Statistics Toolkit

WITHDRAWN

Statistics Toolkit

Rafael Perera

Centre for Evidence-based Medicine
Department of Primary Health Care
University of Oxford
Old Road Campus
Headington
Oxford OX3 7LF

Carl Heneghan

Centre for Evidence-based Medicine
Department of Primary Health Care
University of Oxford
Old Road Campus
Headington
Oxford OX3 7LF

Douglas Badenoch

Minervation Ltd
Salter's Boat Yard
Folly Bridge
Abingdon Road
Oxford OX1 4LB

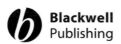
Blackwell Publishing

BMJ|Books

© 2008 Rafael Perera, Carl Heneghan and Douglas Badenoch
Published by Blackwell Publishing
BMJ Books is an imprint of the BMJ Publishing Group Limited, used under licence
Blackwell Publishing, Inc., 350 Main Street, Malden, Massachusetts 02148-5020,
USA
Blackwell Publishing Ltd, 9600 Garsington Road, Oxford OX4 2DQ, UK
Blackwell Publishing Asia Pty Ltd, 550 Swanston Street, Carlton, Victoria 3053,
Australia

First published 2008
3   2012

ISBN: 978-1-4051-6142-8
A catalogue record for this title is available from the British Library and the Library
of Congress.

Set in Helvetica Medium 7.75/9.75 by Sparks, Oxford – www.sparks.co.uk
Printed and bound in Singapore by Markono Print Media Pte Ltd

Commissioning Editor: Mary Banks
Development Editors: Lauren Brindley and Victoria Pittman
Production Controller: Rachel Edwards

For further information on Blackwell Publishing, visit our website:
http://www.blackwellpublishing.com

Contents

This handbook was compiled by Rafael Perera, Carl Heneghan and Douglas Badenoch. We would like to thank all those people who have had input to our work over the years, particularly Paul Glasziou and Olive Goddard from the Centre of Evidence-Based Medicine. In addition, we thank the people we work with from the Department of Primary Health Care, University of Oxford, whose work we have used to illustrate the statistical principles in this book. We would also like to thank Lara and Katie for their drawings.

Introduction

This 'toolkit' is the second in our series and is aimed as a summary of the key concepts needed to get started with statistics in healthcare.

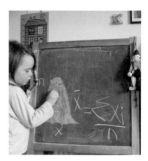

Often, people find statistical concepts hard to understand and apply. If this rings true with you, this book should allow you to start using such concepts with confidence for the first time. Once you have understood the principles in this book you should be at the point where you can understand and interpret statistics, and start to deploy them effectively in your own research projects.

The book is laid out in three main sections: the first deals with the basic nuts and bolts of describing, displaying and handling your data, considering which test to use and testing for statistical significance. The second section shows how statistics is used in a range of scientific papers. The final section contains the glossary, a key to the symbols used in statistics and a discussion of the software tools that can make your life using statistics easier.

Occasionally you will see the GO icon on the right. This means the difficult concept being discussed is beyond the scope of this textbook. If you need more information on this point you can either refer to the text cited or discuss the problem with a statistician.

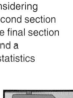

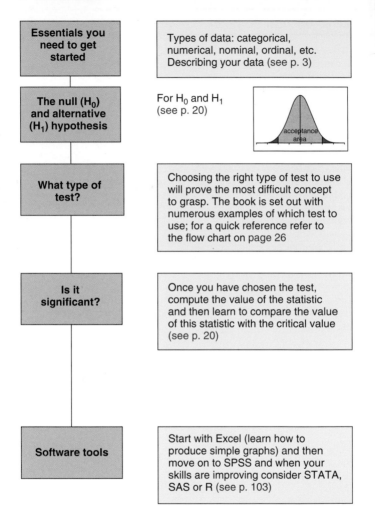

Essentials you need to get started

Types of data: categorical, numerical, nominal, ordinal, etc. Describing your data (see p. 3)

The null (H_0) and alternative (H_1) hypothesis

For H_0 and H_1 (see p. 20)

acceptance area

What type of test?

Choosing the right type of test to use will prove the most difficult concept to grasp. The book is set out with numerous examples of which test to use; for a quick reference refer to the flow chart on page 26

Is it significant?

Once you have chosen the test, compute the value of the statistic and then learn to compare the value of this statistic with the critical value (see p. 20)

Software tools

Start with Excel (learn how to produce simple graphs) and then move on to SPSS and when your skills are improving consider STATA, SAS or R (see p. 103)

Data: describing and displaying

The type of data we collect determines the methods we use. When we conduct research, data usually comes in two forms:

* Categorical data, which give us percentages or proportions (e.g. '60% of patients suffered a relapse').
* Numerical data, which give us averages or means (e.g. 'the average age of participants was 57 years').

So, the type of data we record influences what we can say, and how we work it out. This section looks at the different types of data collected and what they mean.

A variable from our data can be two types: categorical or numerical.

> Any measurable factor, characteristic or attribute is a **variable**

Categorical: the variables studied are grouped into categories based on qualitative traits of the data. Thus the data are labelled or sorted into categories.

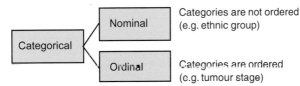

Categorical → Nominal — Categories are not ordered (e.g. ethnic group)

Categorical → Ordinal — Categories are ordered (e.g. tumour stage)

A special kind of categorical variables are **binary** or **dichotomous** variables: a variable with only two possible values (zero and one) or categories (yes or no, present or absent, etc.; e.g. death, occurrence of myocardial infarction, whether or not symptoms have improved).

Numerical: the variables studied take some numerical value based on quantitative traits of the data. Thus the data are sets of numbers.

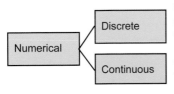

Numerical → Discrete — Only certain values are possible with gaps between these values (e.g. admissions to hospital).

Numerical → Continuous — All values are theoretically possible and there are no gaps between values (weight, height).

You can consider discrete as basically counts and continuous as measurements of your data.

> **Censored data** – sometimes we come across data that can only be measured for certain values: for instance, troponin levels in myocardial infarction may only be detected for a certain level and below a fixed upper limit (0.2–180 µg/L)

Summarizing your data

It's impossible to look at all the raw data and instantly understand it. If you're going to interpret what your data are telling you, and communicate it to others, you will need to summarize your data in a meaningful way. Typical mathematical summaries include percentages, risks and the mean.

The benefit of mathematical summaries is that they can convey information with just a few numbers; these summaries are known as **descriptive statistics**.

Summaries that capture the average are known as measures of **central tendency**, whereas summaries that indicate the spread of the data usually around the average are known as measures of **dispersion**.

The arithmetic mean (numeric data)

The arithmetic mean is the sum of the data divided by the number of measurements. It is the most common measure of central tendency and represents the average value in a sample.

$$\bar{x} = \frac{\sum x_i}{n}$$

Consider the following test scores:

> $\bar{x}$ = sample mean
> μ = population mean
> $\sum$ = the sum of
> x = variable
> i = the total variables
> n = number of measurements

Test scores out of ten

6	4
4	7
5	2
6	9
7	7

2. Divided by the number of measurements
⇓
(6+4+5+6+7+4+7+2+9+7) / 10 = 5.7
⇑   ⇑
1. The sum of the measurements   3. Gives you the mean

To calculate the mean, add up all the measurements in a group and then divide by the total number of measurements.

The geometric mean

If the data we have sampled are skewed to the right (see p. 7) then we transform the data using a natural logarithm (base e = 2.72) of each value in the sample. The arithmetic mean of these transformed values provides a more stable measure of location because the influence of extreme values is smaller. To obtain the average in the same units as the original data – called the geometric mean – we need to back transform the arithmetic mean of the transformed data:

$$geometric\ mean\ original\ values = e^{(arithmetic\ mean\ ln(original\ values))}$$

The weighted mean

The weighted mean is used when certain values are more important than others: they supply more information. If all weights are equal then the weighted mean is the same as the arithmetic mean (see p. 54 for more).

We attach a weight (W_i) to each of our observations (X_i):

$$\frac{W_1X_1 + W_2X_2 + \ldots W_2X_n}{W_1 + W_2 + \ldots W_n} = \frac{\sum W_i X_i}{\sum W_i}$$

The median and mode

The easiest way to find the median and the mode is to sort each score in order, from the smallest to the largest:

Test scores out of ten

1) 2	6) 6	In a set of ten scores take the fifth and sixth values
2) 4	7) 7	⇓
3) 4	8) 7	(6+6) / 2 = 6
4) 5	9) 7	⇑
5) 6	10) 9	The median is equal to the mean of the two middle values or to the middle value when the sample size is an odd number

The **median** is the value at the midpoint, such that half the values are smaller than the median and half are greater than the median. The **mode** is the value that appears most frequently in the group. For these test scores the mode is 7. If all values occur with the same frequency then there is no mode. If more than one value occurs with the highest frequency then each of these values is the mode. Data with two modes are known as **bimodal**.

Choosing which one to use: (arithmetic) mean, median or mode?

The following graph shows the mean, median and mode of the test scores. The *x*-axis shows the scores out of ten. The height of each bar (*y*-axis) shows the number of participants who achieved that score.

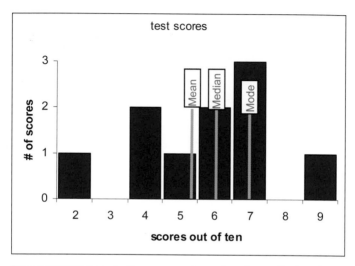

This graph illustrates why the mean, median and mode are all referred to as measures of central tendency. The data values are spread out across the horizontal axis, whilst the mean, median and mode are all clustered towards the centre of the graph.

Of the three measures the mean is the most sensitive measurement, because its value always reflects the contributions of each data value in the group. The median and the mode are less sensitive to outlying data at the extremes of a group. Sometimes it is an advantage to have a measure of central tendency that is less sensitive to changes in the extremes of the data.

For this reason, it is important not to rely solely on the mean. By taking into account the frequency distribution and the median, we can obtain a better understanding of the data, and whether the mean actually depicts the average value. For instance, if there is a big difference between the mean and the median then we know there are some extreme measures (outliers) affecting the mean value.

Distributions

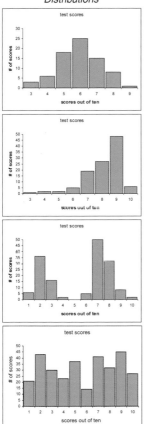

The shape of the data is approximately the same on both the lefthand and righthand side of the graph (symmetrical data). Therefore use the mean (5.9) as the measure of central tendency.

The data are now nonsymmetrical, i.e. the peak is to the right. We call these negatively skewed data and the median (9) is a better measurement of central tendency.

The data are now bimodal, i.e. they have two peaks. In this case there may be two different populations each with its own central tendency. One mean score is 2.2 and the other is 7.5

Sometimes there is no central tendency to the data; there are a number of peaks. This could occur when the data have a 'uniform distribution', which means that all possible values are equally likely. In such cases a central tendency measure is not particularly useful.

Measures of dispersion: the range

To provide a meaningful summary of the data we need to describe the average or central tendency of our data as well as the spread of the data.

> Meaningful summary = central tendency + spread

For instance these two sets of class results have the same mean (5.4)

Class 1 test scores	
4	5
5	6
5	7
5	5
5	4

Mean = 54/10

5.4

Class 2 test scores	
1	6
3	8
3	9
2	6
4	9

However, class 2 test scores are more scattered; using the spread of the data tells us whether the data are close to the mean or far away.

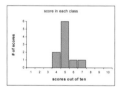
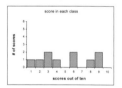

The range for results in class 1 is 4–6   The range for results in class 2 is 1–9

The range is the difference between the largest and the smallest value in the data.

We will look at four ways of understanding how much the individual values vary from one to another: variance, standard deviation, percentiles and standard error of the mean.

The variance

The variance is a measure of how far each value deviates from the arithmetic mean. We cannot simply use the mean of the difference as the negatives would cancel out the positives; therefore to overcome this problem we square each mean and then find the mean of these squared deviations.

> σ^2 = population variance
> s^2 = sample variance

To calculate the (sample) variance:

1. Subtract the mean from each value in the data.
2. Square each of these distances and add all of the squares together.
3. Divide the sum of the squares by the number of values in the data minus 1.

$$s = \frac{\sum (x_i - \overline{x})^2}{n - 1}$$

Note we have divided by $n - 1$ instead of n. This is because we nearly always rely on sample data and it can be shown that a better estimate of the population variance is obtained if we divide by $n - 1$ instead of n.

....

The standard deviation
....

The standard deviation is the square root of the variance:

$$s = \sqrt{\left(\frac{\sum (x_i - \overline{x})^2}{n - 1} \right)}$$

s = standard deviation

The standard deviation is equivalent to the average of the deviations from the mean and is expressed in the same units as the original data.

Consider class 1 results with the mean result of 5.4

x	$x_i - \overline{x}$	$(x_i - \overline{x})^2$
4	−1.4	1.96
4	−1.4	1.96
5	−0.4	0.16
5	−0.4	0.16
5	−0.4	0.16
5	−0.4	0.16
5	−0.4	0.16
5	−0.4	0.16
6	0.6	0.36
7	1.6	2.56

3. Add the squares together

$\sum (x_i - \overline{x})^2 = 7.8$

4. Divide by the number of values n − 1

$\sum (x_i - \overline{x})^2 / n - 1 = 7.8/9 = 0.87$

SD = square root of 0.87 = 0.93

1. Subtract the mean from each value

2. Square each of the distances

Therefore, in class 1 the mean is 5.4 and the standard deviation is 0.93. This is often written as 5.4 ± 0.93, describing a range of values of one SD around the mean.

Assuming the data are from a normal distribution then this range of values one SD away from the mean includes 68.2% of the possible measures, two SDs includes 95.4% and three SDs includes 99.7%.

Dividing the standard deviation by the mean gives us the **coefficient of variation**. This can be used to express the degree to which a set of data points varies and can be used to compare variance between populations.

Percentiles

Percentiles provide an estimate of the proportion of data that lies above and below a given value. Thus the first percentile cuts off the lowest 1% of data, the second percentile cuts off the lowest 2% of data and so on. The 25th percentile is also called the first quartile and the 50th percentile is the median (or second quartile).

Percentiles are helpful because we can obtain a measure of spread that is not influenced by outliers. Often data are presented with the **interquartile range**: between the 25th and 75th percentiles (first and third quartiles).

Standard error of the mean

The standard error of the mean (SEM) is the standard deviation of a hypothetical sample of means. The SEM quantifies **how accurately** the true population mean is known:

$$SEM = s / \sqrt{n},$$

SEM = standard error of the mean

where s is the standard deviation of the observations in the sample.

The smaller the variability (s) and/or the larger the sample the smaller the SEM will be. By 'small' we mean here that the estimate will be more precise.

Displaying data

Most of our graphical displays are about summarizing frequencies making it easier to compare and/or contrast data. They also allow for the identification of outliers and assessment of any trends in the data.

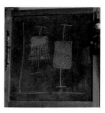

Key elements for the construction of graphs are generally not well understood, which then leads to poor representations and misunderstandings. Commonly graphs generated depend on the statistical package used in the analysis (Excel, SPSS, STATA).

The three key principles of graph construction are:
a) visual detection of data symbols;
b) estimation of values and important relationships;
c) context.

Puhan *et al.* Three key principles of graph construction. *J Clin Epidemiol* 2006;**59**:1017–22.

There are various ways to display your data such as:
- Pie chart
- Bar or column chart
- Histogram
- Stem and leaf
- Box plot
- Dot plot

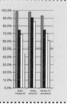

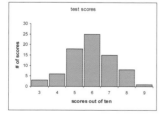

Bar or column chart for test scores: vertical column represents each category with the length proportional to the frequency. The small gaps indicate that the data are discrete.

We used Excel to generate the above bar or column chart.

Use the chart wizard in Excel to get started

Chart type allows you to change the appearance of the display

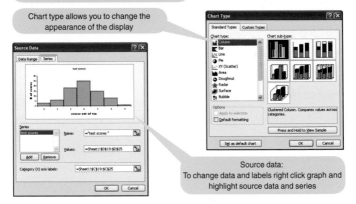

Source data:
To change data and labels right click graph and highlight source data and series

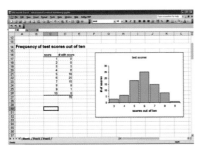

By selecting data series and then selecting options we can reduce the gap width to zero. We now have a **histogram**: similar to the **bar chart** but no gap. This should be used when the data are continuous. The width of each bar would now relate to a range of values for the variable, which may be categorized. Careful labelling should be used to delineate the boundaries.

Pie charts: not often used in scientific papers but can be helpful as visual presentations. The area of the pie segment is proportional to the frequency of that category. Such charts should be used when the sum of all categories is meaningful, i.e. if they represent proportions.
To construct simply select the chart type by right clicking on your chart and select the pie chart icon.

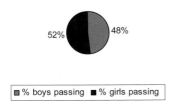

% passes by sex

52% 48%

■ % boys passing ■ % girls passing

Box and whisker plot: is a graphical display of the lowest (predicted) value, lower quartile, median, upper quartile and the highest (predicted) value.

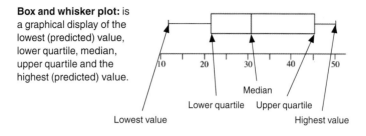

We used SPSS to generate the following box and whisker plot

If the population sampled in your dataset is not normal, you may see many 'outliers' – points outside the predicted lowest and/or highest value.

Dot plot or scatter-plot: used to display two quantitative variables and represent the association between these two variables (this is not the same as causation). Useful for continuous data and correlation or regression.

There are at least four possible uses for scatter-plots:
1) Relationship between two variables (simple).
2) Relationship between two variables graphed in every combination (matrix).
3) Two scatter-plots on top of each other (overlay).
4) Relationship between three variables in three dimensions (3-D scatter-plot).

Probability and confidence intervals

Probability is a measure of how likely an event is to occur. Expressed as a number, probability can take on a value between 0 and 1. Thus the probability of a coin landing tails up is 0.5.

> Probability:
> Event cannot occur = zero
> Event must occur = one

Probability rules

If two events are **mutually exclusive** then the probability that either occurs is equal to the sum of their probabilities.

> Mutually exclusive: a set of events in which if one happens the other does not. Tossing a coin: either it can be head or tails, it cannot be both.

P (heads or tails) = P (heads) + P (tails)

If two events are **independent** the probability that both events occur is equal to the product of the probability of each event.

> Independent event: event in which the outcome of one event does not affect the outcome of the other event.

E.g. the probability of two coin tosses coming up heads:

P (heads and heads) = P (heads) $\times$ P (heads) = 0.5 x 0.5 = 0.25

Probability distributions

A probability distribution is one that shows all the possible values of a random variable. For example, the probability distribution for the possible number of heads from two tosses of a coin having both a head and a tail would be as follows:

- (head, head) = 0.25
- (head, tail) + (tail, head) = 0.50
- (tail, tail) = 0.25

Probability distributions are theoretical distributions that enable us to estimate a population parameter such as the mean and the variance.

> Parameter: summary statistic for the entire population

The normal distribution
The frequency of data simulates a bell-shaped curve that is symmetrical around the mean and exhibits an equal chance of a data point being above or below the mean. For most types of data, sums and averages of repeated observations will follow the normal distribution.

Normal distribution

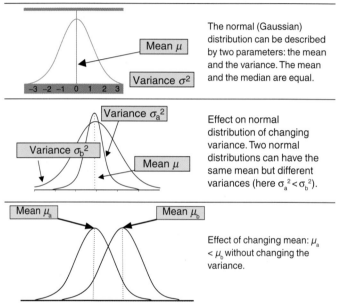

The normal (Gaussian) distribution can be described by two parameters: the mean and the variance. The mean and the median are equal.

Effect on normal distribution of changing variance. Two normal distributions can have the same mean but different variances (here $\sigma_a^2 < \sigma_b^2$).

Effect of changing mean: $\mu_a < \mu_b$ without changing the variance.

Given that the distribution function is symmetrical about the mean, 68% of its area is within one standard deviation (σ) of the mean (μ) and 95% of the area is within (approximately) two standard deviations of μ. Therefore the probability that a random variable x is between:

$(\mu - \sigma)$ and $(\mu + \sigma) = 0.68$ (1 standard deviation)
$(\mu - 1.96\sigma)$ and $(\mu + 1.96\sigma) = 0.95$ (2 standard deviations)

Some practical uses of probability distributions are:
- To calculate confidence intervals for parameters.
- To determine a reasonable distributional model for univariate analysis.
- Statistical intervals and hypothesis tests are often based on specific distributional assumptions.

Underlying the normal distribution is the **central limit theorem**: the sum of random variables have (approximately) a normal distribution. The mean is a weighted sum of the collected variables, therefore as the size of the sample increases, the theoretical sampling distribution for the mean becomes increasingly closer to the normal distribution.

Different distributions: their uses and parameters

Distribution	Common use	Parameters
Binomial distribution	Used to describe discrete variables or attributes that have two possible outcomes, e.g. heads or tails	Sample size and probability of success
The chi-squared distribution	Used with continuous data: inference on a single normal variance; tests for independence, homogeneity and 'goodness of fit'	Degrees of freedom
***F* distribution**	Used for inference on two or more normal variances; ANOVA and regression	Numerator and denominator degrees of freedom
Geometric distribution	Used for modelling rates of occurrence	Probability of event
Log-normal distribution	Used when the data are highly skewed whereas the natural log values of the data are normally distributed	Location parameter and the scale parameter
Poisson distribution	Used for modelling rates of occurrence for discrete variables	The rate (mean)
Student's *t* distribution	Used to estimate the mean of a normally distributed population when the sample size is small. Also for calculating confidence intervals and testing hypotheses	Degrees of freedom

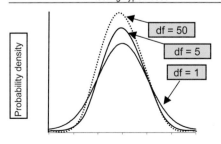

Degrees of freedom (df): the number of observations that are free to vary to produce a given outcome.
Basically how many values would we need to know to deduce the remaining values?
The larger the df the greater the variability of the estimate.

Confidence intervals

Confidence intervals tell you about the likely size of an effect (parameter).

A single guess (estimate) of the mean (our sample mean) does not tell us anything about how sure we are about how close this is to the **true** population mean. Instead we use a range of values – the confidence interval – within which we expect the true population mean to lie. To do this we need to estimate the precision using the standard error of the mean (SEM).

The corresponding 95% CI is:

(Sample mean – (1.96 × SEM) to Sample mean + (1.96 × SEM))

The 95% CI is the range of values in which we are 95% certain the mean lies. When the data is normally distributed but population variance is unknown the sample mean follows a t distribution.

(Sample mean – ($t_{0.05}$ × SEM) to Sample mean + ($t_{0.05}$ × SEM))

This shortens to:

Sample mean $\pm\ t_{0.05} \times \dfrac{s}{\sqrt{n}}$

Where $t_{0.05}$ is the percentage point of the t distribution with $n - 1$ degrees of freedom for a two-tailed probability of 0.05. At this point you need to use a t distribution table. The t distribution produces a wider CI to allow for the extra uncertainty of the sampling.

If we are interested in the proportion of individuals who have a particular characteristic or outcome then we need to calculate the standard error of the proportion SE(p).

$$SE(p) = \sqrt{\dfrac{p(1-p)}{n}}$$

Large standard error = imprecise estimate

Small standard error = precise estimate

The standard error of the proportion by itself is not a particularly useful measure. If the sampling distribution of the proportion follows a normal distribution we can estimate the 95% confidence interval (95% CI) by:

$$P - \left[1.96 \times \sqrt{\frac{p(1-p)}{n}} \right] \quad \text{to} \quad P + \left[1.96 \times \sqrt{\frac{p(1-p)}{n}} \right]$$

The 95% CI is ±1.96 times the standard error of the proportion. This is the most common method used in clinical research that reports the proportion of patients experiencing a particular outcome.

Therefore we could describe the mean of our data and the 95% CI; that is we are 95% confident that the mean lies within this range.

Given that the SE depends on the sample size and the variability of our data, a wide confidence interval tells us the results are imprecise. Also, small samples will give wider CIs than larger samples.

For example, let's say 10 men weigh the following: 95, 97, 98, 99, 94, 97, 95, 96, 92 and 100kg.

Consider the following table and results:

x	$x_i - \bar{x}$	$(x_i - \bar{x})^2$
95	−1.3	1.69
97	0.7	0.49
98	1.7	2.89
99	2.7	7.29
94	−2.3	5.29
97	0.7	0.49
95	−1.3	1.69
96	−0.3	0.09
92	−4.3	18.49
100	3.7	13.69

Mean $(\bar{x})$ = 96.3 kg

$\sum (x_i - \bar{x})^2 = 52.1$

$\sum (x_i - \bar{x})^2 / n - 1 = 52.1/9 = 5.79$

SD = square root of 5.79 = 2.41

Standard error of the mean SEM = $s / \sqrt{n}$ = 2.41/ 3.16 = 0.76 kg

If the SD^2 estimated was equal to the true population variance, then we could calculate the 95% CI using normal distribution =

Sample mean − (1.96 × SEM) to Sample mean + (1.96 × SEM)

96.3 − (1.96 ×0.76) to 96.3 − (1.96 ×0.76)

$$= 94.81 \text{ kg to } 97.79\text{kg}$$

However, generally the true population variance is not known. If we consider the present example, the variance is unknown. We would need to use the *t* distribution to calculate the 95% CI for the true population mean.
Sample mean ± $t_{0.05}$ = 96.3 − (2.262 × 0.76) to = 96.3 − (2.262×0.76)

$$= 94.58 \text{ kg to } 98.02 \text{ kg}$$

Where 2.262 is the percentage point of the *t* distribution with nine df (n − 1) giving a two-tailed probability of 0.05. You can generate the *t* distributions in Excel. Select the Statistical category; select TINV and the screen below will appear.

Probability 0.05

function(fx) feature.

Degrees of freedom

The t distribution

Note now the 95% CI is slightly wider reflecting the extra uncertainty in the sampling and not knowing the population variance. The use of a *t* distribution in this calculation is valid because the sample mean will have approximately a normal distribution (unless the data are heavily skewed and/or the sample size is small).

Hypothesis testing

A hypothesis is an explanation for certain observations. We use hypothesis testing to tell if what we observe is consistent with the hypothesis. Hypothesis testing is fundamental to statistical methods.

In statistics we use the probability of an event occurring to compare two competing hypotheses:

1. Null hypothesis, H_0
2. Alternative hypothesis, H_1

> **Commonly used test of hypotheses:**
> Null hypothesis = no effect
> Alternative hypothesis = there is an effect in either direction

We can use statistical tests to compare these hypotheses. If the probability of the null hypothesis being true is very small, then the alternative hypothesis is more likely to be true. For instance, if we wanted to know about how effective chloramphenicol eye drops are compared with placebo in the treatment of infective conjunctivitis (see p. 25), the hypotheses would be:

   H_0: no effect of chloramphenicol eye drops over placebo
   H_1: eye drops are more or less effective than placebo

If we can reject H_0 then chloramphenicol must have an effect. Notice we have not specified a direction of the effect for the eye drops. The effect could be to make the conjunctivitis worse or better in the children. This is referred to as a **two-tailed test**. For some hypotheses we may state in advance that the treatment effect is specified in one direction: a one-tailed test.

....
The steps in testing a hypothesis
....

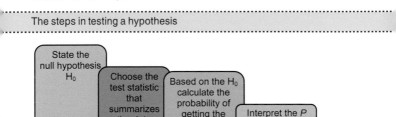

Step 1: It is essential to state clearly your primary null hypothesis and its alternative.

Step 2: Choosing the test statistic is a major step in statistics, subsequent chapters will focus on the most appropriate test statistic to use to answer a specific research question. In addition we have provided flow charts to guide you through the minefield of choosing the appropriate test statistic for your data.

Step 3: Select the level of significance for your test statistic: the level of significance when chosen before the statistical test is performed is called the alpha (α) value.

Conventional values used for α are: 0.05 and 0.01. These values are small because we do not want to reject the null hypothesis when it is true.

> **α value:** the probability of incorrectly rejecting the null hypothesis when it is actually true

Further to this we can use the P value. The P value is the probability of obtaining the result we got (or a more extreme result), if the null hypothesis is true. If you

> **P value:** the probability of obtaining the result if the null hypothesis is true

are having difficulty with this concept then it might be easier to consider the P value as the probability that the observed result is due to chance alone. The interpretation is that if P is small, then what is more likely is that the H_0 is wrong. The P value is calculated after the test statistic is performed and if it is lower than the α value the null hypothesis is rejected.

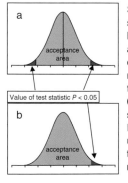

Step 4: Determine the critical value of the test statistic: at what value do we consider the hypothesis proved or disproved? In defining areas of rejection and acceptance in a normal distribution figure, (a) illustrates a two-tailed nondirectional probability distribution. Thus in the blue shaded area the P value is less than 0.05 and we can reject the null hypothesis and say the results are significant at the 5% level. Figure (b) gives an illustration of a one-tailed upper test. If the P value is greater than 0.05 then there is insufficient evidence to reject the null hypothesis.

Step 5: State the appropriate conclusion from the statistical testing procedure.

Errors in hypothesis testing

Type I error: we reject the null hypothesis when it is true. For example, we say that a treatment is beneficial when in fact it isn't.

> The α **value** is the probability of a type I error

Thus to prevent type I errors we set the significance level of the test, the α value, at a low level.

Type II error: we do not reject the null hypothesis when it is false. For example, we think that a treatment is not beneficial when it is. The chance of making a type II error is generally denoted by β.

> The β **value** is the probability of a type II error

The power of a test is the probability of rejecting the null hypothesis when it is false $(1 - \beta)$. Thus high power is a good thing to have because ideally we would want to detect a significant result if it is really present.

Statistical power

In the Rose *et al.* study (see Chapter 5, p. 28) you will see the following in the methods: The initial planned sample size

> **Power = $1 - \beta$**

$(n = 500)$ cited in the original protocol was sufficient to detect this difference with a power of 80%, $\alpha = 0.05$ using a two-tailed test based on a placebo cure rate of 72% and a prevalence of bacterial events of 60%.

After the study is conducted, 'post hoc' power calculations should not be needed. Once the size of the effect is known, confidence intervals should be used to state the likely error of the study estimate.

Factors that affect the power:
1.   Sample size
Power increases with increasing sample size and thus a large sample has a greater ability to detect an important effect.
2.   Effect size
The larger the effect the easier it will be to detect it (higher power).
3.   Significance level
Power is greater if the significance level is larger – the α value is larger. So as the probability of a type I error increases the probability of a type II error decreases (everything else staying equal). So if the α value is changed from 0.01 to 0.05 at the outset then the power of the study increases; increasing the probability of rejecting the null hypothesis when it is true (type 1 error).

Calculating sample sizes:

Different equations are appropriate for different types of data and different types of questions, but sample size calculations are generally based on the following general equation:

$$n = \left(\frac{\text{Two standard deviations}}{\text{Size of effect}} \right)^2$$

For unpaired *t*-tests and chi-squared tests we can use Lehr's formula:

$$\frac{16}{(\text{Standardized difference})^2}$$

for a power of 80% and a two-sided significance of 0.05.

We can try available programs online: for power calculations try the PS program, downloadable free from Vanderbilt University's Department of Biostatistics (http://biostat.mc.vanderbilt.edu/twiki/bin/view/Main/PowerSampleSize).

We could use Altman's nomogram: a nomogram that links the power of a study to the sample size. It is designed to compare the means of two independent samples of equal size. Reproduced from *Br Med J* 1980;**281**:1336–38, with permission from the BMJ publishing group.

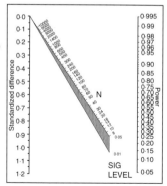

We could use tables: see Machin D. *et al. Sample Size Tables for Clinical Studies,* 2nd edn. Oxford: Blackwell Publishing, 1997.

We could use general formulas, which are necessary in some situations.

Choosing which measure and test to use

Incidence: number of **new** cases in a given time interval

Incidence rate: incidence/number of person time years at risk
Cumulative incidence: incidence/number initially disease free
Hazard rate: number of expected events in instant (time dependent)

Prevalence: number of cases at a given time

Point prevalence: number of cases at one time-point
Period prevalence: number of cases during a period of time

Relative measures: for measuring the ratio of one event or one variable to another

Hazard ratio: the effect of an explanatory variable on the hazard risk of an event
Odds ratio: the ratio of the odds of an event occurring in one group to the odds of it occurring in another group
Relative risk: ratio of the risk of an event occurring in one group to the risk of it occurring in another group
Relative risk reduction: the reduction in the risk made by the intervention compared with the risk of the event in the control group

Absolute measures: for measuring the absolute difference of one event or one variable to another

Absolute risk difference: the difference in the risk for an event between two groups (e.g. exposed vs unexposed populations)

Attributable risk: the proportion of an event in those exposed to a specific risk factor that can be attributed to exposure to that factor

Number needed to treat: the average number of patients who need to receive the intervention to prevent one bad outcome

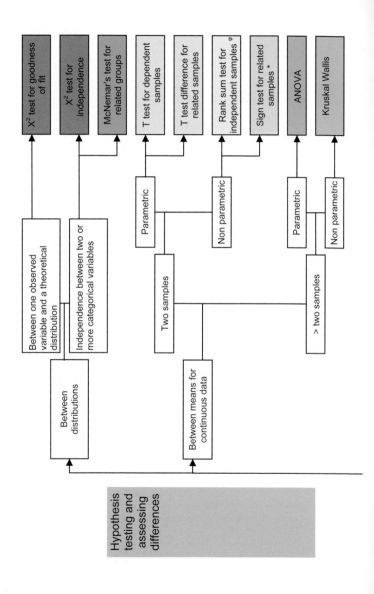

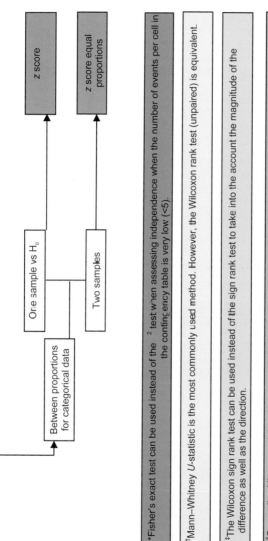

*Fisher's exact test can be used instead of the χ^2 test when assessing independence when the number of events per cell in the contingency table is very low (<5).

†Mann–Whitney U-statistic is the most commonly used method. However, the Wilcoxon rank test (unpaired) is equivalent.

‡The Wilcoxon sign rank test can be used instead of the sign rank test to take into the account the magnitude of the difference as well as the direction.

§Generalized linear models encompass ANOVA, ANCOVA, linear regression, logistic regression and Poisson regression and should be considered when other variables in your data may affect the outcome.

Randomised controlled trials: *mean, median, mode, RD, NNT, Mann–Whitney and log rank tests*

Question: In children with conjunctivitis how effective is chloramphenicol in the treatment of infective conjunctivitis?
Rose *et al. Lancet* 2005;**366**:37–43.

Data were collected on clinical cure at 7 days as stated by parents, microbiological outcomes and further episodes in 6 weeks.

Tests used:
The risk difference (RD) and the **number needed to treat** (NNT) were used for the clinical cure outcome at 7 days. The **Mann–Whitney test** was used to compare time to clinical cure. Clinical cure rates were compared with the **log rank test** and **Kaplan–Meier survival statistics**. Meta-analyses of random-effects models were used to define which bacterial organisms were associated with conjunctivitis, with relative risk as the summary statistic; heterogeneity was assessed by use of the χ^2 and I^2 statistics.

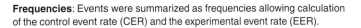

Frequencies: Events were summarized as frequencies allowing calculation of the control event rate (CER) and the experimental event rate (EER).

Risk difference (RD): The main outcome of interest is clinical cure at day 7 – dichotomous: Yes/No. The risk difference provides information on the extra proportion of children who will be cured (by day 7) if treatment is provided.

Proportion cured by day 7 (intention to treat analysis):

$$RD = EER - CER$$

86.4% (chloramphenicol) – 79% (placebo) = 7.4%

95% confidence interval: –0.9% to 15.6%

Which means that chloramphenicol might be as effective as placebo in curing conjunctivitis by day 7.

Numbers needed to treat (NNT): This number gives the average number of children that need to be treated with chloramphenicol to have one extra cured. This is equal to the inverse of the RD (or 1/RD):

$$NNT = 1/RD$$

$$1/7.4\% = 1/0.074 = 13.51$$

The NNT is equal to 14 as it is always rounded up

Relative risk (RR): The ratio of events in the treated group (EER) compared with the control group(CER):

$$\mathbf{RR} = EER/CER = 1.09$$

Relative benefit increase (RBI): The increase on the rates of good events:

$$(EER–CER)/CER = 7.4\%/79\% = 0.09 = 9\%$$

Mann–Whitney test: This method is used to test the hypothesis that the time to clinical cure is the same in both groups. This test is considered a nonparametric test and the reason for its use here is that the time to clinical cure is skewed because most children recover in the first few days of the trial whereas a few others have a prolonged illness lasting several days.

H_0 (hypothesis being tested): The median time to clinical cure in the chloramphenicol group is the same as that in the placebo group.

Example: The Mann–Whitney statistic is calculated from the sum of the ranks and the total number of participants in each group. The number of participants was the same for both arms of the trial = 163, and the sums of the ranks were 24 895 (chloramphenicol) and 28 406 (placebo). These give a mean

> Use the Mann-Whitney test with non-parametric data. Samples need to be independent and the data ordinal or continuous measurements

rank of 152.7 for the chloramphenicol group and of 174.3 for the placebo group. The interpretation is that the placebo group take longer to achieve clinical cure (because their values are on average higher than for those in the chloramphenicol group), with a *P* value of 0.037.

Note: Strictly speaking this method compared the distributions and therefore tests more than whether or not the medians are the same.

Log-rank test and **Kaplan–Meier survival statistics:** If all children (regardless of treatment) recovered within 7 days then measuring those that have recovered at day 7 would show no difference between the groups. Survival methods are used to detect if a difference occurs at a particular time-point in the 7-day period.

Kaplan–Meier curves represent each clinical cure as it happens, whereas the log-rank test is used to test difference between the groups across all time-points.

H_0 **(hypothesis being tested):** The recovery rate over 7 days is the same in the chloramphenicol group and the placebo group.

Log-rank test P value = 0.025

The log-rank test is most likely to detect a difference between groups when the risk of an event is consistently greater for one group than another. In this case the chloramphenicol group recover quicker.

Other statistical methods/terminology used

Meta-analysis was used to test which bacterial organisms are likely causes of conjunctivitis. Three studies that provided information on bacterial growth were combined to give overall estimates (see 'Meta-analysis' and measures of heterogeneity, p. 36). Mean, median and percentages were used to summarise data. Analyses were done using intention to treat whenever possible.

The mean and the median

Means and medians are used in this context to summarise the results for continuous variables. Time to clinical cure (days) is summarised using both types of measurements. The mean (together with the standard deviation) is an excellent descriptor of the central location when the data are symmetrical and, in particular, normally distributed. This is because the mean can be heavily influenced by extreme values. If these are equally likely to happen to the left or to the right of the mean then these balance out. The standard deviation is a good measure of the spread of the data, as long as the mean is an adequate descriptor of the central location, because it is equally affected by extreme measures. The mean time to recovery gives an idea of how long it will take for a child with conjunctivitis who presents to a general practitioner to recover.

> Mean time to recover (standard deviation):
> chloramphenicol: 5.0 days (1.9)
> placebo: 5.4 days (1.9)

The median is always a good measure of the central location of the data; however, it is not as easy to interpret as the mean, and the tests available are also more limited than those for the mean. For that reason it is used generally, instead of the mean, when the data are not symmetrical. As a measure of spread, the interquartile range is given together with the median. Median time to recover (interquartile range):

chloramphenicol: 5 days (3 to 6), placebo: 5 days (4 to 7)

Calculating the mean:

Time to clinical cure – first 15 measurements in placebo group: 6, 4, 1, 3, 5, 2, 6, 5, 0, 7, 3, 7, 3, 5, 7.

The mean is obtained by adding all the recovery times and dividing by the number of children. For the first 15 children this is equal to:

$$6 + 4 + 1 + 3 + 5 + 2 + 6 + 5 + 0 + 7 + 3 + 7 + 3 + 5 + 7 = 64$$

$$\text{Mean} = 64/15 = 4.27$$

Calculating the median:

The median is the number for which half the data is smaller and half larger. The ordered times to recovery for the first 15 children are: 0,1,2,3,3,3,4,**5**,5,5,6,6,7,7,7.

Which means that the 5 (in bold) is the median as it stands in the middle of the ordered set of numbers (in the 8th position).

The risk difference (RD) and the number needed to treat (NNT)

The **risk difference** (also called **absolute risk**) is a measure used to estimate the effect an intervention (or a risk factor) has on the outcome. Chloramphenicol (Ch) is meant to increase the number of clinical cures compared with using placebo (Pl) saline drops. If this is true, then the risk difference should give a measure of the benefit of using this antibiotic.

The risk is the probability of something happening. That 'something' in this case is clinical recovery from conjunctivitis within 7 days. To calculate this probability we use the data obtained from each group in the trial. The number of children that recovered (within 7 days) in the conjunctivitis group was 140 out of 162, whereas for the placebo group it was 128 out of 155. The risk of recovery is then $140/162 = 0.864$, or 86.4%, and $128/155 = 0.826$, or 82.6%, respectively.

Note: The term 'risk' in this case is associated with a positive outcome. This is important as the interpretation of these values depends on this. We look for an increase in risk of a positive outcome, and for a decrease in risk of a negative one.

The risk difference is the difference between the intervention (EER) and the control group (CER):

$$RD = risk\ (Ch) - risk(Pl)$$

$$RD = 0.864 - 0.826 = 0.038 = 3.8\%$$

which means that chloramphenicol increases the chances of recovery by almost 4%. However, we do not know if this is due to chance, so a 95% confidence interval (CI) is required to estimate the potential variation. The 95% CI for the RD is −4.1% to 11.8%, meaning that potentially there is no effect of chloramphenicol compared with placebo.

The **numbers needed to treat (NNT)** is a transformation of the risk difference into the number of people that need to be treated with chloramphenicol to have an extra person cured by day 7. It is the ratio $NNT = 1/RD = 1/0.038 = 26.3$. The NNT is 27 because it is rounded up, and it means that 27 children need to be treated with chloramphenicol to have one extra clinical cure by day 7. In practical terms this is a number commonly used to compare different treatments for the same condition because a small NNT means less people need to be treated to have a clinical cure. One particular drawback to the NNT is that there is no adequate way to calculate its confidence interval (although sometimes it is obtained from the CI of the RD) and therefore it is difficult to assess its uncertainty.

The Mann–Whitney test

Because the time to clinical cure is heavily skewed (most children will recover 'quickly' and a few will have prolonged illness) the usual parametric tests – which assume the data to follow a normal distribution (see p. 16) – are not applicable. The Mann–Whitney test uses the ranks of the times to clinical cure and compares the similarity of these ranks for the chloramphenicol and the placebo groups.

Arm	Ch	Ch	Pl	Pl	Pl	Ch	Ch	Ch
Day to cure	7	5	1	4	6	3	7	6
Arm	Pl	Pl	Pl	Pl	Ch	Pl	Ch	Ch
Day to cure	1	8	4	8	4	6	8	3

Which would give the following ranks to the data:

Arm	Ch	Ch	Pl	Pl	Pl	Ch	Ch	Ch
Rank	12.5	8	1.5	6	10	3.5	12.5	10
Arm	Pl	Pl	Pl	Pl	Ch	Pl	Ch	Ch
Rank	1.5	15	6	15	6	10	15	3.5

Of note is that whenever there are several children with the same duration they all receive the same rank. For example, there are two children that recovered within 1 day; because the ranks they would receive would have been 1 and 2 they both get the average rank, 1.5. The sum of these ranks is then used to check if the difference in them would be equal to that expected by chance or not. For this example the sums of the ranks are:

Sum of ranks Ch = 12.5 + 8 + 3.5 + 12.5 + 10 + 6 + 15 + 3.5 = 71
Sum of ranks Pl = 1.5 + 6 + 10 + 1.5 + 15 + 6 + 15 + 10 = 65

This is compared (subtracted) to the expected sum of ranks, which is equal to $N^*(N + 1)/2$ where N is the number of participants in each group (N can be different for each group).

Mann–Whitney Ch = $71 - (8 \times 9/2) = 35$
Mann–Whitney Pl = $65 - (8 \times 9/2) = 29$

The largest statistic – in this case 35 – is then used to calculate the P values, usually from Mann–Whitney tables or statistical software packages. In this case the P value is equal to 0.75, meaning that both groups appear to have the same median time to clinical cure (for these 16 data points).

Log-rank test and Kaplan–Meier survival statistics

The proportion of children that have not recovered is calculated every time a clinical recovery is reported. In this study these can only occur each day (the outcome was measured using diaries) and hence the daily steplike shape. To calculate the Kaplan–Meier estimates, the total number that recovered is divided by those that are still being followed-up. This corrects for those that drop out during the trial. Those children for whom no recovery date has been recorded are counted as being censored (because the length of their illness is unknown). These appear as crosses in the graph and could happen at any point during the study. For example, a child that had not recovered by day 7 and for whom no further information was available (but still ill) would appear as a cross at day 7 and would not be included in the calculation for day 8.

The log-rank test statistic is obtained by comparing the observed recoveries and those expected if both groups behaved the same. This test is also called the Mantel–Cox χ^2 test.

Kaplan–Meier curves

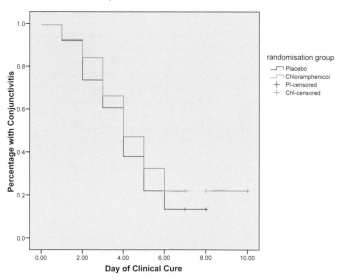

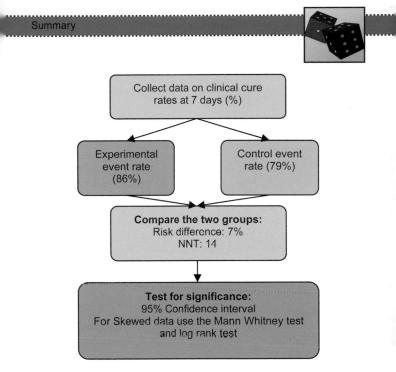

Collect data on clinical cure
rates at 7 days (%)

Experimental
event rate
(86%)

Control event
rate (79%)

Compare the two groups:
Risk difference: 7%
NNT: 14

Test for significance:
95% Confidence interval
For Skewed data use the Mann Whitney test
and log rank test

Systematic reviews 1: odds, odds ratio, heterogeneity, funnel plots

Question: In patients on anticoagulation with warfarin, does self-monitoring or self-management lead to improved outcomes?
Heneghan *et al. Lancet* 2006;**367**:404–11.

The purpose of systematic reviews is to combine all of the unbiased studies that have been done on a particular question. If the review can pool the individual data from each of these studies (a meta-analysis), it can greatly increase the statistical power of the research by treating them as if they were in one large sample instead of many small ones.

When we read systematic reviews, we are principally concerned with:
- whether the review found and included all the good-quality studies;
- how to extract and pool the data from different studies; and
- whether it makes sense to combine them.

The reviewers found 14 RCTs and extracted data on thromboembolic events, major bleeding, death and the proportion of measurements that were within the target range.

The review reports the setting, follow-up, sample size and intervention details for each study included.

> **Tests used: The odds ratio** (OR) was used to calculate a combined measure from all of the studies: three different methods were employed.
>
> The data were tested for **heterogeneity** using the χ^2 and I^2 statistics. Two tests were used to detect for **publication bias**: Begg's rank correlation and Egger's linear regression.

Using odds to represent risk:

The risks of clinical events were presented as the **odds** of the event in each group. The odds is the ratio of the number of patients that have the event to the number of patients that do not have it. If 10 people have a heart attack out of 100 in the intervention group the odds are 10/90 = 1:9. Note the difference between the odds and frequencies: frequencies in the same group = 10/100 = 10%.

What are odds?
Odds are a way of stating the probability of an event. When we look at a group of patients, the odds of the event in that group are the number of patients who have an event divided by the number who do not.

	Control group	Experimental group
Event	A	B
No event	C	D

The odds of an event in the control group is A/C; likewise, the odds of an event in the experimental group is B/D.

Menendez Jandula 05, from Heneghan *et al. Lancet* 2006;**367**:404–11.

Odds of thromboembolic event in the control group 20/(369 − 20)

$$20/349 = 0.057$$

Odds of thromboembolic event in experimental group = 4/(368 − 4)

$$4/364 = 0.011$$

This might seem like a convoluted way of doing things, but odds have particular statistical properties that lend themselves to meta-analysis.

Odds ratios

When we want to compare the difference between a control and experimental group, we can use the odds ratio (OR). The OR is the ratio of the odds in one group divided by the odds in a different group: the experimental group's odds divided by the treatment group' odds.

Menendez Jandula 05, from Heneghan *et al. Lancet* 2006;**367**:404–11.

Experimental group odds: 0.011

Control group odds: 0.057

$$OR = 0.011/0.057 = 0.19$$

95% confidence interval: 0.06 to 0.57

If the odds ratio is greater than one, it indicates more events in the experimental group; if it is less than one, it indicates fewer events in the experimental group. If the odds ratio is exactly one, there is no difference between the groups. If the confidence interval around the odds ratio overlaps the value of one, we can say that it is not statistically significant.

....
Combining odds ratios
....

In this review, the authors used a fixed effects model to combine the odds ratios into one overall estimate. Where heterogeneity existed in the data, they used a random effects model.

In a systematic review, we don't just want to compare the odds between one control group and one experimental group; we want to combine lots of data from different control and experimental groups.

Unfortunately, we can't just add up all the participants on each side (this would break the randomisation potentially giving the wrong results): to retain the validity of the original research, we have to work with the odds ratios from each study and not the total numbers of patients.

The easiest way to do this would be to take the mean of all the odds ratios. However, this would give the same weight to all studies regardless of the number of participants (meaning that each patient would count double in a study containing 100 participants compared with one containing 200). We need to take into account that some studies provide more information than others (e.g. higher event rates).

Therefore, when we combine odds ratios we have to adjust for the study size and event rate. The **standard error (SE)** is a statistical measure that takes both of these factors into account. It is commonly assumed that the smaller the **SE** in a study's results, the more importance the study should be given.

> The inverse of the square of the standard error (SE) gives a measure of precision; the larger the precision around any measure, the more certain we are of the measure itself.

There are two approaches to combining the studies, based on the types of assumption made about the nature of the data:

1. Fixed effects model: The fixed effects model is based on the assumption that all the different data sets come from the same population and are measuring the same thing. In other words, the 'true' treatment effect in each study is in fact identical.

> Use the Mantel–Haenszel approach when it is safe to assume that the data are from similar studies and have moderate sample sizes.
>
> Use the Peto method when there are very low event rates.

In this review, the Mantel–Haenszel approach was used. This approach assumed a fixed effect model, which gives greater weight to odds ratios from studies with a lower standard error.

Unfortunately, some statistics perform less well in different circumstances. When event rates are very low or zero in some groups, the Peto method is useful. In this review, the authors verified their findings using the Peto method.

2. Random effects model: The random effects model assumes that each study is measuring something different. Its purpose is to obtain the average for the distribution of the effects of the individual studies.

The random effects model usually results in a more conservative estimate of the combined odds ratio (i.e. the confidence interval will be wider, indicating less certainty as to the true value).

> Use the DerSimonian–Laird random effects model when there is some evidence of heterogeneity amongst the data.

However, although their underlying assumption is more reasonable, random effects methods are considered less robust than fixed effects methods. The reason is that the former give more weight to smaller trials, which tend to be of lower quality.

Usually, reviewers will carry out both types of analysis (fixed and random effects): if they are consistent, that is good news.

One way to tell whether the fixed effect model assumption applies is to look at the data and see how much variation, or heterogeneity, there is. The reviewers in this study tested their data to see if they were heterogeneous; where this was the case, they used a random effects model instead.

Heterogeneity tests

Our main concern in conducting systematic reviews is whether it is valid to combine the data. If (and only if) we are satisfied that the clinical and methodological characteristics of the studies are similar, can we examine the data to see if they are consistent.

Of course, we would expect some variation, through statistical chance and through differences in the baseline risk of the different populations.

So, the aim of statistical homogeneity tests is to test the hypothesis that the data are similar between studies and that it makes sense to combine them.

The **chi-squared (χ^2) test for homogeneity** is such a test. Use it when you have a set of measurements and you want to know the probability that they are more different from one another than you would expect by chance. The test produces three important numbers: the chi-squared statistic, the degrees of freedom and the P value.

> Use chi-squared when you have a set of measurements and you want to know the probability that they differ from one another more than you would expect by chance variation.

As a rule of thumb, if the chi-squared statistic is greater than the degrees of freedom, there is evidence of heterogeneity. When the P value is given, this rule of thumb is not necessary. If the P value is small, this indicates that the studies are unlikely to be homogeneous.

However, chi-squared P values are very sensitive to the number of values being tested, and there is some controversy about the validity of this heterogeneity test in meta-analysis.

This is where the **I-squared (I^2) statistic** comes in. I^2 describes the percentage of total variation across the data that is due to heterogeneity rather than chance and is more stable than the χ^2 statistic for homogenity. The result is given as a percentage, with large values representing large heterogeneity.

Visualising statistical significance

Forest plots are used to display all of the results for a given intervention and outcome in a graphic form. This makes is easy for the reader to get a feel for the spread of the data, and to see how much uncertainty there is around the results.

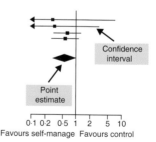

This example is shown from the lower half of Figure 2 in the paper. The small squares represent the odds ratio for each individual study that looked at thromboembolic events in patients who were self-monitoring (testing but not adjusting their anticoagulation therapy).

The horizontal line through each square shows the confidence interval around that study's odds ratio. Presenting the results in this way enables us to tell straight away whether the results are statistically significant. In this example, none of the four individual studies is statistically significant alone because each crosses 1 (no effect).

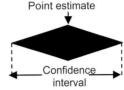

Point estimate

The diamond is used in a similar way
to show the combined odds ratio and confidence
intervals for the meta-analysis.

Confidence
interval

In this example, the confidence interval
does not cross 1 – the 'line of no difference',
so the meta-analysis has found a statistically significant result.

Note that it is essential to report the numbers for the odds ratio and confidence intervals as well.

Three points to remember about forest plots:

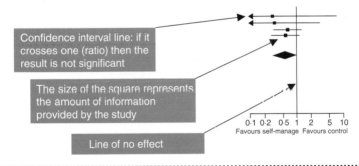

Confidence interval line: if it crosses one (ratio) then the result is not significant

The size of the square represents the amount of information provided by the study

Line of no effect

0.1 0.2 0.5 1 2 5 10
Favours self-manage Favours control

Subgroup analysis

Subgroup analyses are meta-analyses on subgroups of the studies. They are used to test the hypothesis that different settings (e.g. primary or secondary), different patient characteristics (e.g. age) or different ways of delivering care (e.g. dosage) might affect the outcomes.

In this review, the reviewers set out to analyse subgroups of studies according to their patient characteristics (mechanical valve replacement or atrial fibrillation), and the type of self care used (self-monitoring or self-adjusted therapy).

The authors also carried out a post hoc analysis, which means that they decided to look at this factor after they had collected the data. Post hoc analyses are to be treated with caution because they are far more likely to be 'false positives' from chance patterns appearing in the data than a priori analyses.

There are problems and limitations with using subgroup analysis, which can result in misleading conclusions:

- To reduce the possibility of finding a significant result by chance the number of subgroups should be kept to a minimum.
- All analyses should be prespecified to minimize spurious findings.
- There should be a rationale for all subgroup analyses.
- That difference between subgroups may be due to other confounding factors that have not been identified.

Meta-regression: Meta-regression investigates whether particular covariates – trial specific characteristics like drug dose, duration of training, etc. – explain any of the heterogeneity of treatment effects between studies.

 Thompson SG, Higgins JP. How should meta-regression analyses be undertaken and interpreted? *Stat Med* 2002;**21**(11):1550–73.

Testing for publication bias

Many researchers have found that studies with positive, significant results are over-represented in the literature compared with studies with negative or nonsignificant results.

In this review, publication bias was investigated using a funnel plot. This technique involves plotting the precision of studies against their point estimate result. The usual method, used in this review, is to use **standard error** (of the log of the odds) to represent study precision and the **log of the odds ratio** for the point estimate.

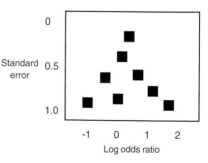

If the meta-analysis is valid, more precise studies should show less variation in their results than less precise ones. This gives rise to the funnel shape shown opposite.

If the shape is asymmetrical, it may be because some negative studies are missing from the review because of publication bias.

Two tests were used to examine whether there was significant publication bias.

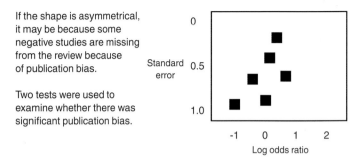

Egger's linear regression test
Egger's regression test is often used to help detect publication bias in meta-analyses. For funnel plot asymmetry: Egger's tests for the Y intercept = 0 from a linear regression of normalized effect estimate (estimate divided by its standard error) against precision (reciprocal of the standard error of the estimate).

Egger M, Davey Smith G, Schneider M, Minder C. Bias in meta-analysis detected by a simple, graphical test. *Br Med J.* 1997;**315**:629–34.

Begg's rank correlation test: tests for the interdependence of variance and effect size using Kendall's method. This method makes fewer assumptions than Egger's test. However, it is insensitive to many types of bias to which Egger's test is sensitive. Thus unless there are many studies in the meta-analysis, the Begg method has very low power to detect such bias.

Begg CB, Mazumdar M. Operating characteristics of a rank correlation test for publication bias. *Biometrics* 1994;**50**:1088–101.

Sensitivity analysis is repeating the analysis to see if omitting some studies, including others, or changing some assumptions, makes a difference to the results. This was used to investigate whether low quality studies (which we might expect to be biased in favour of self-monitoring).

Individual patient data analysis (IPD):

An IPD meta-analysis includes collecting specific individual data from the randomised trials in the systematic review. An intention to treat analysis is performed, assessing clinical and statistical heterogeneity. Multilevel models with patients and trials as the two levels can be explored to investigate treatment effect on various outcomes.

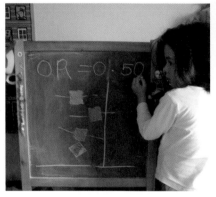

Simmonds MC *et al*. Meta-analysis of individual patient data from randomized trials: a review of methods used in practice. *Clin Trials* 2005;**2**(3):209–17.

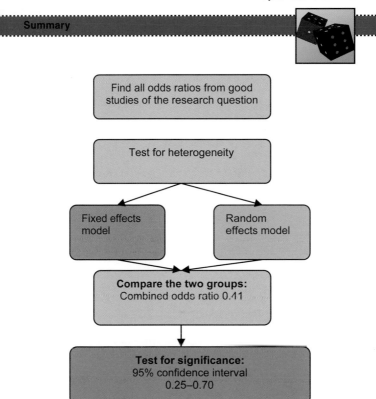

Find all odds ratios from good
studies of the research question

Test for heterogeneity

Fixed effects
model

Random
effects model

Compare the two groups:
Combined odds ratio 0.41

Test for significance:
95% confidence interval
0.25–0.70

Use Cochrane RevMan for your analysis; this is free to download from the
Cochrane Collaboration Information Management System website
(http://www.cc-ims.net/RevMan/download.htm).

The *Cochrane Handbook for Systematic Reviews of Interventions* (formerly
the *Reviewers' Handbook*) is available on the Cochrane Collaboration website
(http://www.cochrane.org/resources/handbook/).

Case-control studies: odds ratios, logistic regression

Question: What are the effects of parenteral penicillin for children with meningococcal disease (MD) before hospital admission in preventing morbidity and mortality?
Harnden *et al. Br Med J.* 2006;**332**(7553).

Data were collected on death and complications in survivors.

> The effects of penicillin and other factors were considered with adjustment of **crude odds ratios** done by **logistic regression**.

Case-control study: The data in this study were collected by identifying children that died from meningococcal disease (MD) (cases) and selecting similar children in terms of age and location (controls) who survived a meningococcal infection. On average 1 in 10 children with MD die, while the number of controls per case in this study was roughly 4 to 1. One reason for using this design is to have enough 'cases' in the study; this strategy is used particularly if the condition is rare.

Odds ratios (OR): One statistic used to summarise if a factor – in this case administration of parenteral penicillin by general practitioners – is associated with the event of interest – death – is the odds ratio.

> The odds ratio compares the chances (odds) of death in those that did not receive penicillin with the chances (odds) of death in those that did.

Calculating odds ratios: data taken from Harnden et al.

Penicillin odds: A/C: 22/83 = 0.265

Control odds: B/D: 2/45= 0.044

	Exper. Penicillin	Control
Event	A	B
No event	C	D

Odds of dying

OR = A/C / B/D = 5.96
95% confidence interval: 1.34 to 26.52

This means that penicillin increases the chances of a child dying by a factor between 1.3 to 26.5 times the initial levels.

GO

Logistic regression: Although the cases and controls were matched by age and region, there is potential for confounding. One way confounding might work is that those children who are more severely ill will be more likely to be diagnosed with meningococcal disease and therefore given penicillin. If this is the case we would expect that more of the children in the penicillin group will die compared with the non-penicillin group, because the latter group would be less severely ill.

A confounding variable is one that affects the results of your study.

Logistic regression aims to 'adjust' for this potential confounding by fitting a model that uses all other possible factors (such as serogroup C infection, haemorrhagic rash, septicaemia, time to admission, etc.) that could have an effect on mortality. The result of this model is a series of odds ratios (one for each explanatory factor) that take into account the effect of all other factors on mortality at the same time. This group of odds ratios are usually called '**adjusted odds ratios**' because they adjust for those confounders included in the model (but **only** for those included in the model).

Table 6.1 Odds ratios from logistic regression model

Factor	Adjusted odds ratio (95% CI)
Male	1.86 (0.66 to 5.12)
Penicillin given before admission	7.45 (1.47 to 37.67)
Serogroup C infection	4.12 (1.53 to 11.08)
Onset to admission <25th centile	1.29 (0.42 to 3.89)
GP assessed illness as severe	1.83 (0.66 to 5.12)
Haemorrhagic rash before admission	0.66 (0.14 to 3.09)
Septicaemic disease without localisation	2.68 (0.73 to 9.86)
Oral antibiotics in week before admission	2.16 (0.30 to 15.55)

This means that combining all the available factors gives only two that appear to increase mortality. These are having a serogroup C infection, and being given penicillin before hospital admission. All other factors have confidence intervals that include 1, meaning that the odds of dying potentially do not increase (or decrease) by, for example, having a haemorrhagic rash before admission.

In particular, the adjusted odds ratio for penicillin given before admission increased to 7.4 (95% CI 1.5 to 37.7). This would mean that either the penicillin does increase mortality, or that there is still confounding present that has not been corrected by the available data.

Odds ratios in case-control studies

Odds ratios are one of the most commonly used statistics in medicine. As their name indicates they are the ratio of two odds. Odds are not the same as probability. A probability or proportion is obtained from those that have the event out of the total number of people. In this example the proportion of children that died out of those given penicillin is the number that died (22) out of the total that were given penicillin (105).

Proportion that were given penicillin and died = 22/105 = 0.21 = 21%

On the other hand the odds of dying if given penicillin are obtained from the ratio of those that died and those that survived in the penicillin group.
Odds dying if given penicillin = 22/83 = 0.265

> Proportion = 22/105 = 0.21 = 21%
> Odds = 22/83 = 0.265

Although this appears as a proportion it is not, if we think of the event as surviving, then the odds of surviving if given penicillin would be 83/22 = 3.77, which is clearly not a proportion. In fact the odds can be any number between 0 and infinity (if the denominator is equal to 0).

The odds ratio in this example compares the odds of dying if given penicillin versus dying if not given penicillin:

> Odds dying if not given penicillin = 2/45 = 0.044
> Odds ratio (OR) = (22/105)/(2/45) = 5.96

If the odds ratio is equal to 1 it means that the odds are the same for both groups. If it is larger (smaller) than 1 then it means that the odds of dying are higher (lower) in the penicillin group. An odds ratio of 5.96 means that giving penicillin to children increased the chances of dying almost six-fold.
Odds ratios are commonly used because they can be calculated regardless of the type of study carried out. In this instance, the use of a (matched) case-control study meant that the calculation of a relative risk is not feasible because there are many more deaths in the group collected than what would be expected by following all children with meningococcal disease in the UK.

Using a contingency table to calculate the odds ratio:
A table (usually two rows and two columns) is often used to show the relationship between disease and exposure.

	Disease +ve	Disease −ve
Exposure	A	B
No exposure	C	D

If we want to know whether exposure to the potential cause is more likely amongst those with the disease than amongst those without it, the odds ratio can be calculated as $(a \times d)/(b \times c)$

An OR >1 shows that the exposure was more common in those with the disease than without; an OR <1 shows that it was less common.

The further interpretation of the OR in a case-control study will depend on the way the information has been obtained. These interpretations are outside the scope of this book, but a good and clear discussion can be found in Kirkwood B, Sterne J. *Essential Medical Statistics,* 2nd edn. Oxford: Blackwell Science, 2003 .

Logistic regression and adjustment for crude odds ratios

Logistic regression is a statistical model that is used to describe whether the chances of an event happening – in this case death – increase, decrease, or are not affected by other factors such as age, sex, presence of signs and symptoms, type of infection, etc.

This type of regression differs from linear regression in that the outcome being modelled is dichotomous (dead/alive), whereas for linear regression it would be continuous.

One simple way to describe this model is the following formula:

$\ln(\text{OR of dying}) = B0 + (B1 \times \text{factor1}) + (B2 \times \text{factor2}) + \dots + (B8 \times \text{factor 8})$

ln = natural logarithm
B0 = intercept
B1, B2… = slope factor 1, 2…
OR = odds ratio
SE = standard error

Thus the natural log of the odds ratio of dying is equal to the sum of the log odds ratios of all the possible contributory factors.

The use of ln (natural logarithm, $\ln(2.72) = 1$) here is due to the fact that the logarithm of the odds ratio behaves very much like a normal continuous variable (this is also exploited when obtaining its 95% confidence interval, see below).

As we can see from the formula, all factors are included at the same time in the model. The B1, B2, etc. relate to the increase (if positive) or decrease (if negative) in the logarithm of the odds ratio of dying associated with the factor. In the model, the Bs provide the odds ratios for each factor when all other factors are being taken into consideration and therefore receive the name of **adjusted estimates of the logarithm of the odds ratio**. To obtain the adjusted odds ratios the Bs are transformed to the odds ratio scale using the exponential function, which is the inverse of ln. OR dying (factor 2) = exp(B2)

The values shown in Table 6.1 are exactly these odds ratios obtained from a model that included as factors possibly associated with death: penicillin given before admission, serogroup C infection, onset to admission <25th centile, GP assessed illness as severe, haemorrhagic rash before admission, septicaemic disease without localisation, and oral antibiotics in week before admission. All of these are associated with an increase in the chances of dying except for presenting with a haemorrhagic rash (only OR < 1). This might sound surprising until we remember that only children with MD were included in the study; which meant the chances of having a haemorrhagic rash were much higher than for the overall population.

To decide if the associations are due to chance we must look at the confidence interval for each odds ratio. In this case, having a serogroup C infection and being given penicillin before hospital admission are the only factors where this association is probably not due to chance.

Note: Although in this paper logistic regression was used, the fact that the cases and controls were individually matched by age and region means that the appropriate method for analysis would have been **conditional logistic regression**. This is because we would expect the matched controls to behave more like the case they are matching than to other cases. The results using conditional logistic regression were not presented as it would have meant losing some children from the sample (a few cases did not have matching controls) and the results for both methods were almost the same (no difference in the interpretation).

The information obtained in any study is always an approximation of what is happening in real life (at a population level): generally, the larger the study, the better the approximation. Therefore all statistics obtained will be an approximation, and we need somehow to describe the uncertainty associated with each finding. One way to do this is to present confidence intervals for each of these statistics.

A **confidence interval** refers to a range of values where we expect the real population measure to be. In this example, the confidence interval given for the odds ratio of dying if given penicillin before hospital admission goes from 1.27 to 38.50. This would mean the **real (population) odds ratio** should be a value between these two numbers.

When describing a confidence interval a percentage is always mentioned. Most commonly this is 95%; 95% confidence intervals are reported in the majority of articles, and this is the one reported above. This percentage relates to how confident we are about the chances of the interval created containing the population value. Other common choices for confidence intervals are 90% and 99%. As these percentages increase so does the length of the confidence interval.

> For this example we have the following confidence intervals:
> 90% CI: 1.70 to 20.87
> 95% CI: 1.34 to 26.52
> 99% CI: 0.84 to 42.39

There are different methods to calculate confidence intervals; however, the one most commonly used is the approximation to the normal distribution.

In this method, the statistic used – for example the OR – can be thought of as having approximately a normal distribution. If this is the case, then the 95% CI is obtained as the

> The log(OR) approximates a normal distribution, while the OR does not.

point estimate minus (plus) 1.96 times the standard error of the estimate for the lower (upper) limit.

The 1.96 comes from the fact that within this value 95% of the values in the standard normal distribution would be contained.

For this example:
$$OR = 5.96 \text{ and the } \ln(OR) = 1.79$$
$$\text{and the } SE[\log(OR)] = 0.76$$

95% CI for the log(OR):

Lower limit	$\ln(OR) \pm 1.96 \times SE[\log(OR)]$	$1.79 - (1.96 \times 0.76) = 0.29$
Upper limit		$1.79 + (1.96 \times 0.76) = 3.28$

The 95% CI for the OR is the exponential of the limits obtained above:
Lower limit: $\exp(0.29) = 1.34$
Upper limit: $\exp(3.28) = 26.52$

Summary

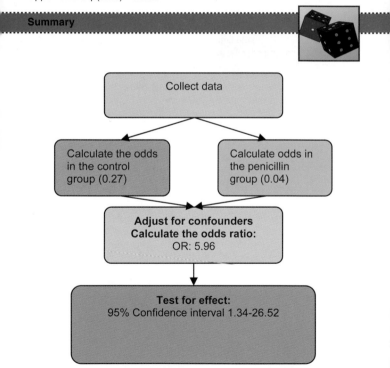

Collect data

Calculate the odds in the control group (0.27)

Calculate odds in the penicillin group (0.04)

Adjust for confounders
Calculate the odds ratio:
OR: 5.96

Test for effect:
95% Confidence interval 1.34-26.52

Questionnaire studies 1: weighted mean frequency, nonparametric tests

Question: In children what are the early clinical symptoms and signs of meningococcal disease?
Thompson *et al. Lancet* 2006;**367**:397–403.

Data were collected on symptoms including the time of day of onset using a checklist.

> A weighted mean frequency was used. Nonparametric bootstrapping was done to calculate 95% CIs around the mean frequencies.
>
> The onset of illness was taken as the time when the parents noticed the first symptom. The time at which each subsequent symptom developed was then calculated from the time of illness onset, rounded to the nearest hour. The median time of onset and interquartile range for each symptom were used.

Weighted mean frequency

The frequency of signs and symptoms for meningococcal disease were obtained using all cases of meningococcal disease (MD) as reference. The mortality rates were used for this, which gave the weights applied for the frequencies found in deaths and in survivors. This weighted frequency is an estimate for the frequency of the sign or symptom in children with meningococcal disease.

Freq all = [freq deaths × mortality rate] + [freq surv × (1 – mortality rate)]

Freq (leg pain) = [22.3% × 6.8%] + [37.7% × 93.2%] = 36.7%

Nonparametric bootstrapping for 95% CI

A 95% confidence interval gives a measure of the variability of the weighted frequency. To obtain this while accounting for the extra deaths in the sample, a technique called bootstrapping was used. Simulations of the data with the correct proportions of deaths and survivors provide the distribution for frequency, which is then used to calculate a lower and upper limit for the 95% CI.

Frequency of leg pain – 95% confidence interval:
Lower limit = 28%
Upper limit = 47%

Median and interquartile ranges

The median is a very stable measure of the centre of the data that is hardly affected by extreme values (at either end of the scale). Measuring the time until a symptom appears is subject to having some extreme cases; for example, one child presenting with leg pain many hours after the start of the illness. For this reason the median was chosen to represent the centre of the data and the interquartile range chosen to give a measure of the spread, instead of the standard deviation.

Weighted mean frequency

There are several situations when the groups represented in a dataset should not be treated equally. The aim was to obtain information on the frequency of each of the symptoms and signs in meningococcal disease because specific ones that occur frequently might aid early diagnosis. However, simply obtaining the frequency in the dataset would be misleading, because the study design means that deaths are over-represented when compared with the real-life situation (the population).

A cohort study that followed children over time would give information on the proportion of children with meningococcal disease and how many of these died. However, such a study would be highly impractical because meningococcal disease is relatively rare compared with other conditions.

By obtaining information on deaths in children and then matching these deaths to a number of survivors, the study artificially sets the ratio of deaths to survivors. The actual rate of deaths is high in children with meningococcal disease (6–12%) but this is much lower than the 33% used in the dataset.

Weighted means are a way of giving more 'importance' to different groups in the data. In this case it was a way of standardising the information recorded in the data to that found in the population. The weights are generally chosen to reflect how important we expect each group to be. An example of a similar situation can be found when using meta-analysis to give importance to different trials in the dataset (see p. 36).

From population studies in the UK we know that the mortality rate for the age group studied is around 6.8%. This means that out of 1000 children with meningococcal disease, 68 will die and the rest will survive:

```
                                          ➤ 68 die
1000 children with meningococcal disease ⟨
                                          ➤ 932 survive
```

The frequency of a particular symptom might be different in those that died and those that survive. To obtain the frequency in the population (regardless of survival status) we take into account the frequency for each group and combine them using weights.

$$\text{Overall frequency} = 36.7\% \begin{cases} 0.068 \times 22.3\% \\ 0.932 \times 37.7\% \end{cases}$$

The weight of 0.068 comes from 68/1000.

....
Nonparametric bootstrapping was done to calculate 95% CIs
....

Bootstrapping is a technique that uses simulation and is very popular mainly because of its flexibility. In its nonparametric form (most commonly used) it consists of assuming the data – a sample from the population – to be equivalent to the population and generating samples (with replacement) from it. For example, if the data consisted of 10 children that had the following result for leg pain:

Child	1	2	3	4	5	6	7	8	9	10
Pain	N	Y	N	N	N	Y	Y	N	Y	Y

Random samples of any size can be generated from these data by allowing replacement; that is allowing each child to appear more than once in a sample. Here are five samples of size 5 generated from the data. Note: using the same approach, larger samples can also be obtained.

Samples generated: Frequency

Child	2	8	1	5	1
Pain	Y	N	N	N	N

1/5

Child	3	3	8	8	9
Pain	N	N	N	N	Y

1/5

Child	6	8	5	9	8
Pain	Y	N	N	Y	N

2/5

Child	2	1	5	5	3
Pain	Y	N	N	N	N

1/5

Child	8	3	10	8	1
Pain	N	N	Y	N	N

1/5

The statistic of interest – in this case the frequency of the symptom – can be obtained from each sample, and assuming that the original data are representative of the population, a histogram of the statistic of interest obtained from all the samples should be roughly equivalent to the distribution of the statistic. In other words, the simulations give a good representation of the variability in the statistic of interest, in this case the frequency.

With this in mind, obtaining confidence intervals is straightforward.
This is done by ordering results from the simulations (smaller to larger). If we have enough simulations, we should see a normally distributed set of results, as illustrated below. We can use these data to work out where the lower and upper 95% CI limits would lie.

In the article, 1000 samples were generated through simulation. The limits for the 95% CI would be (after ordering) the 25th and 975th frequency for the lower and upper limits, respectively.

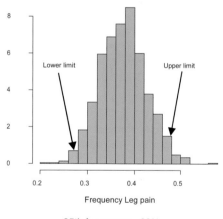

Frequency Leg pain

25th frequency = 28%
975th frequency = 47%

The 95% confidence interval for the frequency of leg pain = 28 to 47%.

This method was used because the dataset had a much larger number of deaths than would be expected in the normal population. The samples in the simulations accounted for this by sampling from both groups – survivors and deaths – according to the mortality rate seen in the population. So the probability that a child that died was included in the sample was equal to the mortality rate, while for a survivor it was (1 – mortality rate).

The median time of onset and interquartile range

The definition of a median is that value that separates the data in half – with (roughly) 50% on either side. The median does not have the same mathematical properties as the mean, but is very stable (in statistical terms this is usually called robust).

For this reason, the median is commonly used when describing data that are likely to have an asymmetrical shape. This generally means that comparatively large values are more common than small ones (or vice versa).

In the case of reporting the time to onset of leg pain, there were a total of 41 children in the age group 1–4 years of age. This sign usually appears moderately early in the disease (75% of the children that present this sign do so within 13 hours). However, in some cases it takes very long to appear – one after 70, one after 79 and one after 96 hours. The mean would give a distorted view of the onset of this symptom. By calculating the median, these extreme values do not affect our estimation of the centre. If these extreme cases had presented values of 700, 760 and 960 hours, or 37, 38 and 39 hours (the next largest value is 36), the results using the medians would not have been affected.

In the same way, the standard deviation is not a good measure of spread because it suffers from the same problems as the mean. To give an estimate of the spread it was decided to use the interquartile range: that is, the range between the 3rd quartile or 75th percentile (value that separates the data with 75% below it, and 25% above it) and the 1st quartile or 25th percentile (separates the data with 25% below it, and 25% above it).

Time from onset of disease to appearance of leg pain in children between 1 and 4 years of age:

Median (or 2nd quartile): 6 hours
1st quartile: 0 hours
3rd quartile: 13 hours

Interquartile range: 0–13 hours

Note: In difference to a 95% confidence interval, the median can be equal to one of the extremes in the interquartile range, meaning that at least 25% of the data points have the same value as the 1st and 2nd quartiles.

Summary

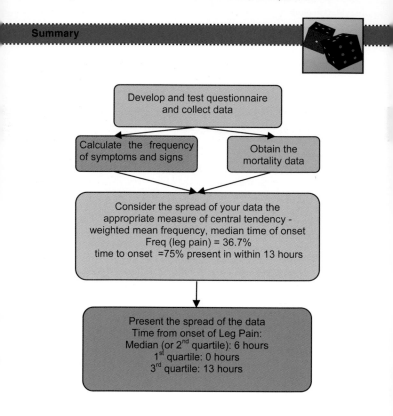

Questionnaire studies 2: inter-rater agreement

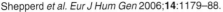

Question: What are the criteria needed to assess the quality of information produced for the public on genetic screening and testing?

Shepperd *et al. Eur J Hum Gen* 2006;**14**:1179–88.

Data were collected on items of information on genetic testing and/or screening for selected genetic conditions. Each item was rated using a **Likert scale**.

Data were analysed using a measure of **inter-rater agreement**. **Kappa** with quadratic weights was used to assess for the level of agreement.

Likert scale

A five-point Likert scale (1, 2, 3, 4, 5) with anchors 1 = 'no, the criteria has not been filled' and 5 = 'yes, the criteria has been filled', was used to rate each item in the scale. The aim here was to create a valid score; what matters is not the actual value recorded for each item but whether the values were reliable.

Inter-rater agreement

The main aim of this paper was to create criteria that could be used to assess the quality of information on genetic screening and testing. For this, groups of experts were asked to identify the different elements that should be included. An important aspect of these elements is that they should be reliable – that is, that different people with similar background should give a similar rating to the same object. High reliability indicates that these criteria are meaningful and usable as valid measures. This is called the level of **inter-rater agreement**, and in the case of categorical or ordinal values is generally measured using a **kappa statistic**.

Kappa statistic

The kappa statistic was used to measure the level of agreement between raters for each one of the different elements evaluated as part of the criteria. Twenty-three questions were considered for inclusion, and the kappa statistic used to determine which ones would be most valuable. Questions with the lowest kappas were discarded or merged with other related questions. Of the 19 that made it to the final criteria, the ones with the lowest kappa values were 'Aims achieved' and 'Local information' with a - $\kappa = 0.25$. The question with the largest kappa was 'Psychological consequences', - $\kappa = 0.75$. This would mean that the inter-rater agreement for the different questions varied between fair and good. There were no 'excellent' items, and the ones that were 'poor' were excluded from the criteria.

Likert scales

A Likert scale is probably the most commonly used scale in questionnaires. It is used when the answer to a question has two extreme positions (e.g. strongly disagree vs strongly agree) and where there is a gradient between these (e.g. mildly disagree, neutral, mildly agree).

There are several types of Likert scales: 3-point, 4-point, 5-point and 7-point, with the 5-point scale being the most popular. The results from this scale are ordinal, which means that statistical methods for their analysis are usually nonparametric ones (e.g. Mann–Whitney), while medians, modes and interquartile ranges are used to summarise these data.

Is risk explained in simple terms?

No				Yes
1	2	3	4	5

Likert scale

In this paper, Likert scales were used to measure the quality of the information on genetic screening. The higher the value for each one of these questions, the better the quality of the information. There were several questions proposed as each one addressed different aspects of the information provided such as the clarity of the aims, clear explanations about the condition, treatment and management choices, etc.

Assessing inter-rater agreement using kappa

Inter-rater agreement can be measured in different ways. For categorical and ordinal data, a kappa statistic is normally used. Other measures like proportional agreement and correlation have been proposed, but these do not measure agreement. In the case of proportional agreement, high levels could be attained by simply guessing; correlation measures linear association, which means that there might be no agreement and perfect correlation (and it is not appropriate for categorical outcomes).

Cohen's kappa is a measure of agreement that corrects for chance agreement. Agreement that occurs by chance (Pc) can be thought of as the agreement you would expect if the rating was done completely at random. This chance agreement is then compared with the observed agreement (Po), which is the actual agreement rate. The kappa score is then calculated using the following formula:

$$Kappa = (Po - Pc)/(1 - Pc)$$

As the maximum value that the observed agreement can attain is 1, this means that when there is perfect agreement the kappa score will be equal to 1. A kappa of 0 would mean that the observed agreement is equal to the expected one, that is, virtually no real agreement. Finally, kappa values can also be negative if the observed agreement is less than that expected by chance. This basically would mean that the raters are in disagreement, and usually a value of 0 is reported instead.

To explain how to calculate a kappa let's imagine the following setup. There are two raters and a number of children (N) examined by both and classified as having (Yes) or not having (No) the disease.

OBSERVED

		Rater 1		
Rater 2		Yes	No	
Yes		A	B	$A+B$
No		C	D	$C+D$
		$A+C$	$B+D$	N

From these data we can create a table of what would be expected if the agreement was equal to that found by chance. The margins of the table will remain the same whereas the values inside each cell would be recalculated as the expected numbers.

EXPECTED

		Rater 1		
Rater 2		Yes	No	
Yes		$(A+B) \times (A+C)/N$	$(A+B) \times (B+D)/N$	$A+B$
No		$(C+D) \times (A+C)/N$	$(C+D) \times (B+D)/N$	$C+D$
		$A+C$	$B+D$	N

We can calculate the observed rate of agreement as the sum of the values within the cells with [Yes, Yes] and [No, No] in the 'Observed' table divided by the total number of children (N). The expected rate of agreement can be obtained using the same method but from the 'Expected' table.

Observed agreement = P_o   **Expected agreement = P_c**

$P_o = (A+D)/N$ $P_c = ((A+B)\times(A+C) + (C+D)\times(B+D))/N^2$

Finally the kappa measure is obtained from these agreement rates:

Kappa = $P_o - P_c/(1 - P_c)$

Example: Here is an example of two raters (GP1 and GP2) and their kappa after measuring 100 children with a URTI (upper respiratory tract infection) and rating them as having a bacterial infection or not.

OBSERVED

GP 2	GP 1 Yes	No	
Yes	35	10	45
No	5	50	55
	40	60	100

EXPECTED

GP 2	GP 1 Yes	No	
Yes	$(45 \times 40)/100$	$(45 \times 60)/100$	45
No	$(55 \times 40)/100$	$(55 \times 60)/100$	55
	40	60	100

Observed agreement = P_o   **Expected agreement = P_c**

$P_o = (35 + 50)/100 = 0.85$ $P_c = (45 \times 40) + (55 \times 60)/100^2 = 0.51$

Kappa = $(0.85 - 0.51)/(1 - 0.51) = 0.69$

A kappa value above 0 means that the agreement was higher than that expected by chance. The following table gives a guideline for the interpretation of different values of kappa.

Interpretation

Value of kappa	Strength of agreement
<0.20	Poor
0.21–0.40	Fair
0.41–0.60	Moderate
0.61–0.80	Good
0.81–1.00	Very good

Which would mean that for the above example with a $\kappa = 0.69$, the strength of agreement would be rated as good.

Kappa statistics can also be used to measure agreement for ordinal scales. In these cases, disagreements are given 'marks' depending on how close they are, for example:
* perfect agreement gets 1 mark;
* one category out gets 0.5 marks;
* two categories out gets 0.25 marks.

The kappa calculated using these marks is called a weighted kappa for obvious reasons. The calculation of the expected agreement and the observed agreement follows the same principles as the previous example (obtained from an Observed table and an Expected table) with the addition of those near agreements with their given weights.

The following is an example of a weighted kappa where the two GPs are now rating 100 children as being not ill (A), moderately ill (B) or severely ill (C).

Observed	GP1			
GP2	A	B	C	Total
A	27	2	3	32
B	4	30	5	39
C	2	2	25	29
Total	33	34	33	100

Expected		GP1		
GP2	**A**	**B**	**C**	**Total**
A	10.56	10.88	10.56	32
B	12.87	13.26	12.87	39
C	9.57	9.86	9.57	29
Total	33	34	33	100

The following table shows the agreements 0 away [(A,A), (B,B), (C,C)], 1 away [(A,B), (B,A), (B,C), (C,B)], and 2 away [(A,C), (C,A)]:

Weights

	Observed	Expected	Weights	Obs × wi	Exp × wi
0	82	33.39	1	82	33.39
1	13	46.48	0.5	6.5	23.24
2	5	20.13	0.25	1.25	5.0325
Total	100	100		89.75	61.662

$$\text{Kappa} = (0.90 - 0.62)/(1 - 0.62) = 0.74$$

These data show good agreement between GP1 and GP2.

Likert scales were used for the evaluation of each question. Because this is an ordinal scale, weighted kappas were obtained. The questions with the lowest kappa were 'Aims achieved' and 'Local information' with a - $\kappa = 0.25$; meaning that their agreement was only 'fair'. The largest kappa obtained was for the 'Psychological consequences' question - $\kappa = 0.75$; meaning that the level of agreement for this question was 'good'.

Summary

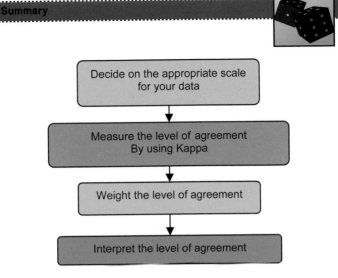

Decide on the appropriate scale
for your data

Measure the level of agreement
By using Kappa

Weight the level of agreement

Interpret the level of agreement

Cohort studies: prevalence, incidence, risk, survival, mortality rate, association, prognostic factor

Question: In men with untreated prostate cancer, what are the expected outcomes after 10 years of survival?
Johansson *et al. JAMA* 2004;**291**:2713–19.

The purpose of population-based cohort studies is to understand the natural history and progression of disease. Prospective, longitudinal cohort studies offer the best method for understanding these factors over a long period of time, principally because they reduce potential 'lead time' bias.

The researchers in this example wished to study the progression of prostate cancer beyond 10 years of survival. Their objective was to explore the association between patients' clinical features and disease progression: does the presence of a particular prognostic factor predict disease progression or death in the future?

This is particularly relevant in diseases such as prostate cancer:
- most sufferers die with prostate cancer rather than of it;
- although early intervention does not affect 5–10-year survival, it may be that men with a longer life expectancy would benefit from treatment.

Prognostic factor: A prognostic factor is any clinical feature that is associated with a particular disease outcome in the future. A prognostic factor can be considered the same as a risk factor.

> **Tests used: Mortality rates**, in terms of events per 1000 patient years, were used to represent disease progression.
> Calculate a combined measure from all of the studies. Three different methods were employed.
>
>
>
> **Poisson** and **linear regression models** were used to test the association between specified **prognostic factors** and disease progression.

Progression-free survival: One type of measurement that can be used in a study to help determine whether a new treatment or exposure is effective. It refers to the probability that a patient will remain alive, without the disease getting worse.

Mortality rates: The proportion of the population in the study: in this case men with prostate cancer that die during a specified period (20 years).

$$\text{Rate} = \frac{\text{Number of events that occurred}}{\text{Total number of years of follow-up for all individuals}}$$

Using mortality or survival rates

Measuring survival time is useful, but it is even better if we can assess the event rates as related to time, because this will give us a more objective picture of what is going on.

Events per 1000 patient years =

$$\frac{\text{Total number of events}}{\text{Total follow-up years} \times 1000}$$

Divide the number of events by the total amount of time the patients were followed (events per 1000 patient years)

We might question the use of events per 1000 patient-years as a statistic in this instance, because most of the participants were followed up to the end of their lives. Events per patient might be more useful.

The main benefit of patient-years as the denominator is in circumstances where we can only follow patients for a relatively short period of their lives.

	Progression of prostate cancer	Death from prostate cancer
Events	39	35
No. of patients	223	223
Mean follow-up	21 years	21 years
Patient-years	$21 \times 223 = 4683$	$21 \times 223 = 4683$
Events per patient-year	39/4983 = 0.00832	35/4983 = 0.00747
Events per 1000 patient-years	8.3	7.4

Data from Table 2 in Johannsen *et al.*

Note that the authors measured observed survival and progression-free survival by applying these methods to different outcomes.

Expected survival:

Relative survival was estimated by comparing the patients' survival statistic with an 'expected' survival for a disease-free population. In order to do this, the authors estimated the expected survival using the **Hakulinen method**, which gives age-adjusted survival rates.

Brenner, Hakulinen On crude and age-adjusted relative survival rates. *J Clin Epidemiol* 2003;**56**:1185–91.

Regression: are the outcomes associated with prognostic factors?

In this study, the authors wanted to know whether and by how much the outcomes were associated with a range of variables:

1. Duration of follow-up
2. Age
3. Grade of tumour
4. Stage of disease

To do this, they needed to deploy one of the most frightening phrases in biostatistics: multivariate analysis, using regression models.

The purpose of regression models is to test the hypothesis that an association exists between an outcome and a potential cause or risk factor.

Use Poisson when: modelling rates or counts

Use linear regression when: modelling continuous outcomes

In statistical terms, the events (or response variable) you want to measure may be predicted by another factor, or (independent) variable.

Use logistic regression when: modelling binary outcomes

Not only can multivariable analysis tell you this, but also it can tell you whether it does so independently from any other.

Poisson regression models

Poisson models are so called because of the distribution of the data: they are not normal!

Use the Poisson regression model when one of the variables is a count (such as an event rate).

Interpreting multivariable analysis

The hard part of multivariable analysis is working out which approach to use; the results are comparatively easy to interpret:

1. Relative risk (see p. 29) for the group of patients with that risk factor.
2. Confidence interval.

(see p. 29)

Summary

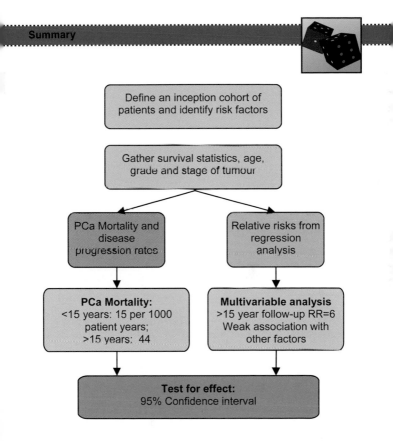

Define an inception cohort of patients and identify risk factors

Gather survival statistics, age, grade and stage of tumour

PCa Mortality and disease progression rates

Relative risks from regression analysis

PCa Mortality:
<15 years: 15 per 1000 patient years;
>15 years: 44

Multivariable analysis
>15 year follow-up RR=6
Weak association with other factors

Test for effect:
95% Confidence interval

Systematic reviews 2: Cohort study odds ratios and relative risk

Question: How well does B-type natriuretic peptide predict death and cardiac events in patients with heart failure?
Doust *et al. BMJ* 2005;**330**(7492):625.

Data were collected on the relationship between measurements of B-type natriuretic peptide (BNP) and the risk of death, cardiac death, sudden death or cardiovascular events.

Tests used: Cox proportional hazards model, relative risk, odds ratio and the hazard ratio.

The purpose of this study was to evaluate the use of BNP as a prognostic factor for heart failure. That is, does BNP predict subsequent heart failure?

Prognostic factors
When we want to predict an event in a group of patients, there is no 'control' group against which to compare outcomes. Therefore, prognostic studies need to compare the risk of events between different subgroups of patients. Typically those that have a factor (or more of it if continuous) vs those that do not.

Remember that in prognostic studies, it is essential that:
- Participants are recruited at a similar point in the course of the disease
- Outcome measures are objective
- Outcome measurements are blind to assessments of prognostic factors

In this case, the subgroups we are interested in are defined by the BNP measurements.

So, in prognostic studies we are testing the hypothesis that the outcome could be predicted by the patient's BNP level – higher BNP, higher risk.

Regression models
Because there may be lots of different factors, some studies test the hypothesis that heart failure could be caused by any one of them.

For this approach, a special kind of regression – a Cox proportional hazard model for the hazard ratio – is used. The key thing to understand here is that this model will show which factors (sometimes only one or none) are the most robust predictors of the outcome.

Because the study was a systematic review, the authors used meta-analysis to combine data from all the different studies included in the review.

Hazard ratio

The first step is to establish the risk of heart failure. This was done using the hazard rate.

Hazard ratio is similar to the relative risk (see p. 29), in that it tells you the proportional increase (or decrease) in the risk of an outcome in one group compared with another. It differs from the relative risk in terms of how it is calculated. The relative risk can be seen as the ratio of two cumulative risks up to a given point in time, for example after 6 months or after 1 year. On the other hand, the hazard is a measure of the risk at that instant (not cumulative). The hazard is normally expressed as a function (over a given period of time) and the hazard ratio would be the ratio of two functions - not of two values as is the risk ratio.

Cox proportional hazards model

Because the hazard is a function over time, in some instances we can assume that the ratio of two hazards remains constant over that period. What this means is that even though the hazard changes over time – e.g. the chances of dying increase as you grow older – in relative terms the ratio of the hazards – those with high BNP vs those with low BNP level – remains constant over time.

The advantage of this setup is that it is not necessary to define what the hazard function is because we are only interested in how this hazard changes given a particular factor – we are only interested in the hazard ratio. These models are given the name of **Cox proportional hazards models** (as Cox was the first one to suggest it).

If the assumption of proportional hazards is valid (as with any model, all assumptions made need to be validated) then the interpretation of the hazard ratio obtained is simple. It tells of the effect that the factor has in increasing (if the hazard ratio is greater than 1) the risk. For this review the estimated increase per 100 pg/mL is of 35% (95% CI 22–49%), meaning that the chances of dying increase by over a third per each 100 pg/mL difference in BNP independent of other factors.

Summary

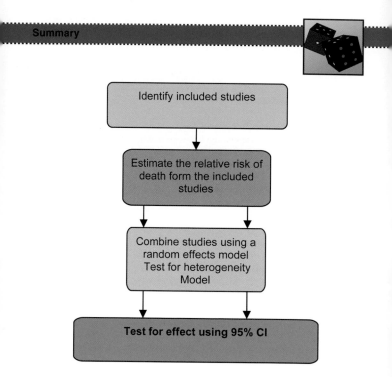

Diagnostic tests: sensitivity, specificity, likelihood ratios, ROC curves, pre- and post-test odds, pre- and post-test probability

Question: In children with suspected influenza, does near patient testing perform as well as laboratory testing in identifying the disease?
Harnden et al. *BMJ* 2003:**326**:480.

The purpose of studies that evaluate diagnostic tests is to compare their performance against a 'gold standard of diagnosis'. To do this, they must:

Gold standard: aims to provide a definitive diagnosis of a condition; however, sometimes not practical or possible

- recruit a cohort of patients similar to those in which the test would be used in real life;
- perform both the experimental test and gold standard test on the cohort of patients;
- ensure that the two sets of test results are evaluated blind to each other.

In this study, the authors recruited children from primary care who were suspected of having influenza.

The tests were evaluated using the following statistical measures:
- **sensitivity**
- **specificity**
- **likelihood ratio**

Statistical significance was tested using **95% confidence intervals**.
Test performance at different 'cut-off' points may be explored using **receiver-operator characteristic (ROC)** curves.

There are four possible outcomes when we perform a diagnostic test with a dichotomous result:

1. True positive
2. False positive
3. False negative
4. True negative.

Dichotomous: divided or dividing into two sharply distinguished parts or classifications

This can be represented in a 2 × 2 table:

	Disease positive	Disease negative
Test positive	a	b
Test negative	c	d

The ideal test would have zero patients in cells *c* and *b*. That is, 100% sensitivity and 100% specificity.

How well does the test detect the disease?

We want to know how likely it will be that a test will correctly identify a patient's disease state. This means considering the columns in the 2x2 table (the patients who had the disease and the patients who didn't)

Sensitivity: is the proportion of people with disease who have a positive test. In the 2 × 2 table, calculate as: $a/(a + c)$.

Specificity: is the proportion of people free of disease who have a negative test. In the 2 × 2 table, calculate as: $d/(b + d)$.

These are usually reported as percentages. Note that a study may have high c but proportionally low b.
In this example, we have the following figures:

	RT-PCR disease positive	RT-PCR disease negative
Near-patient test positive	27	3
Near-patient test negative	34	93

Sensitivity = 27/(27 + 34) = 0.44 or 44%
Specificity = 93/(93 + 3) = 0.97 or 97%

This test has a high specificity; that is, there are very few false positive results. The test would therefore be useful to 'rule in' the disease, if a positive result is found.

How likely is a given test result to be true?

We can also consider whether a particular test result is accurate.

Positive predictive value (PPV) is the proportion of patients who test positive who actually have the disease. In the table, calculate as: $a/(a + b)$

Negative predictive value (NPV) is the proportion of patients who test negative who genuinely don't have the disease. In the table calculate as: $d/(c + d)$

The PPV and NPV statistics are less useful because they will give different results with different levels of prevalence. Sensitivity and specificity will be the same whatever the prevalence.

Likelihood ratios (LR)

It is useful to combine a measure of how much information is provided by a given test result, regardless of prevalence.

This is the likelihood ratio. It is the ratio of the probability that a given test result would occur in a patient with the disease to the probability that the same result would occur in a patient without the disease.

Thus, the LR works on the columns of the 2×2 table, and is therefore independent from disease prevalence, yet gives a measure of test efficacy that applies to a specific test result.

For a positive test result:
sensitivity/(1 – specificity)
=   0.44/0.03 = 14.7

$$LR+ve = \frac{a/(a + c)}{b/(b + d)}$$

For a negative test result:
(1 – sensitivity)/specificity
=   0.56/0.97 = 0.578

$$LR-ve = \frac{c/(a + c)}{d/(b + d)}$$

As a general rule of thumb:
- an LR of 10 or more can rule in a diagnosis;
- a LR of 0.1 or less can rule out a diagnosis.

However, this rule breaks down when the prevalence of the disease is very low.

....

What about tests that have a range of possible results?

....

It is often the case that a diagnostic test does not yield a dichotomous positive/negative result. Rather, we may have a range of values, each of which is to be validated against an objective and definitive assessment of disease status.

In these circumstances, likelihood ratios can be calculated in the same way as before. Thus, for a five-category set of test results, the calculations would be as shown below:

Serum ferritin	Disease positive	Disease negative
Level 1	a	b
Level 2	c	d
Level 3	e	f
Level 4	g	h
Level 5	i	j

So, for a result in the range of level 2 or above:

$$LR2 = \frac{((a + c)/(a + c + e + g + i))}{((b + d)/(b + d + f + h + j))}$$

....

Measuring test performance at different cut-off points

....

The latter approach can be extended to methods of exploring what would be the best 'cut-off' point for defining 'positive' and 'negative' test results.

Consider the above example. If we defined 'Level 2 or 1' as being the range of a 'positive' test result, the test would have the following characteristics:

$$\text{Sensitivity: } (a + c)/(a + c + e + g + i)$$
$$\text{Specificity: } (b + d)/(b + d + f + h + j)$$

If we were interested in a test that had few false negatives (i.e. had high sensitivity), we could define levels 1, 2 and 3 as being 'positive':

$$\text{Sensitivity: } (a + c + e)/(a + c + e + g + i)$$

Specificity: $(b + d + f)/(b + d + f + h + j)$

Of course, setting the threshold lower would be likely to yield more false positive results, that is, increased sensitivity would come at a price of lower specificity.

This process is useful, however, in working out what is the optimum cut-off point for defining positive and negative results. By calculating sensitivity and specificity for different test results we can plot the performance of the test in a **receiver operator characteristics (ROC)** curve:

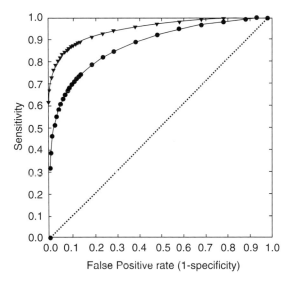

The curve plots sensitivity against (1 – specificity); the closer the curve is to the top left corner (i.e. the closer both sensitivity and specificity are to 1 at the same time), the better its performance.

In this example, two different tests are compared; this yields both a quick visual assessment of the tests and a precise method of comparing them quantitatively, by measuring the area under the curves.

Statistical significance

Confidence intervals should be reported around
each of the measures of diagnostic efficacy.

The key question in interpreting CIs, because there is no 'line of no
difference', is 'Would I interpret the results in the same way at the lower end
of the CI as at the higher end?'

Pre-test odds and post-test odds: particularising the evidence

It is possible to use the likelihood ratio to particularise the results for an
individual patient.

The likelihood ratio is a type of odds ratio; therefore we have to use pre-test
and post-test odds.

Pre-test odds = $(a+c)/(b+d)$
In this example: $(27 + 34)/(3 + 97) = 0.61$

Once a given test result has come back for a particular patient, the post-test
odds can be worked out by multiplying the pre-test odds by the likelihood
ratio. Thus, for a positive test result:

Post-test odds = Pre-test odds $\times$ LR+

In this example: $0.61 \times 0.97 = 0.59$

Converting between odds and percentages
Odds can be converted to and from a percentage or absolute risk (as long as
it is a probability; that is, between 0 and 1) using the following formulae:

Percentage = Odds/(Odds + 1)

Odds = Percentage/(1 − Percentage)

This is particularly useful when you wish to see how informative the test result
is at different levels of pre-test probability. Fortunately, there are numerous
tools to help you do this, particularly the likelihood ratio nomogram and
CATmaker: download at the Centre for Evidence-Based Medicine website
(www.cebm.net).

Using Bayes theorem and the Fagan nomogram

Bayes theorem

The posterior probability is proportional to the prior probability multiplied by a value; the likelihood of the observed results.

The pre-test probability of the disease reflects the prevalence of the disease (or other prior information). In this case 39% of children were RT-PCR positive $(a+c)/(a+b+c+d) = 61/157$

LR = 14.7

Draw a straight line on the nomogram from 39% through the LR of 14.7 and then read off the post-test probability, approximately 90%

The post-test probability is thus the probability that the patient has the disease given a positive test result. The nomogram can also be used for the negative test result.

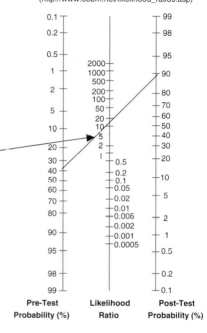

Nomogram for converting Pre-test Probabilities to Post-test Probabilities for a diagnostic test result with a given Likelihood Ratio.
(http://www.cebm.net/likelihood_ratios.asp)

Pre-Test Probability (%)   Likelihood Ratio   Post-Test Probability (%)

Perera R, Heneghan C. Making sense of diagnostic test likelihood ratios. *ACP J Club* 2007;**146**(2):A8--9.

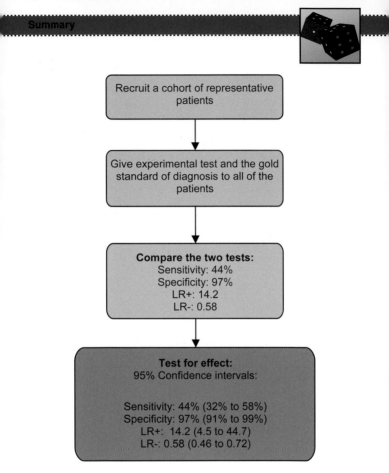

Recruit a cohort of representative patients

Give experimental test and the gold standard of diagnosis to all of the patients

Compare the two tests:
Sensitivity: 44%
Specificity: 97%
LR+: 14.2
LR-: 0.58

Test for effect:
95% Confidence intervals:

Sensitivity: 44% (32% to 58%)
Specificity: 97% (91% to 99%)
LR+: 14.2 (4.5 to 44.7)
LR-: 0.58 (0.46 to 0.72)

Scale validation: *correlation*

Question: Is a measure of severity recorded by a parent equivalent to that recorded by a health practitioner? What are the characteristics that a scale requires to be valid?

Shepperd *et al. J Clin Epidemiol* 2004;**57**(8):809–14.

Data were collected on children with an upper respiratory infection to determine their illness severity as measured by nurses, doctors and parents. This was done using a **visual analogue scale**. A scale that measures functional severity and burden to the parents called CARIFS (Canadian Acute Respiratory Illness and Flu Scale) was also used as outcome and compared with the other measures of severity.

> **Correlations** were used to determine if parental measure of severity is equivalent to severity measured by a health practitioner. The internal consistency of the CARIFS score was assessed using **Cronbach's alpha statistic**.

Visual analogue scale (VAS)

Data obtained from these scales are treated as a continuous variable. It can be any number, usually between 0 and 10. In this study the VAS was used as a measure of severity, with 0 equal to 'best possible health' and 10 equal to 'worst possible health'.

Spearman rank-correlation coefficient (ρ)

Measures of severity of illness in children were obtained from nurses, doctors and parents using visual analogue scales. For parents, a scale called CARIFS was also obtained. This last scale is composed of three different dimensions – symptom presentation, burden on function, and parental impact. Spearman rank-correlations were used to determine if there is good association between parental measurements and those obtained from health professionals (doctors and nurses).

	CARIFS					
	Overall	*P. impact*	*Function*	*Symptom*	*GP VAS*	*Nurse VAS*
GP *VAS*	0.13	0.09	0.03	0.16	–	–
Nurse *VAS*	0.35	0.20	0.38	0.36	0.24	–
Parent *VAS*	0.40	0.29	0.36	0.41	0.09	0.23

These values show that there is a very small correlation between measurements by the GP and by the parent, that is, there is no good agreement about the child's severity, with the highest level of agreement found between CARIFS symptom dimension and the GP (VAS) score. Other measurements show a better association, the highest being parent assessment of severity using VAS and their recording of the presence of symptoms for an upper respiratory infection.

Crohnbach's alpha

This measures how consistent the items in a scale are. This is important because the scale is meant to measure severity of illness as assessed by the parent. Values of alpha between 0.6 and 0.9 are deemed to be adequate. The alpha value obtained for these data was 0.85, which would mean that the overall scale has good internal consistency.

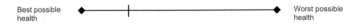

Visual analogue scale and CARIFS

A visual analogue scale is just another name for a line with two anchors at either end.

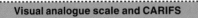

Best possible health   Worst possible health

A respondent would then draw a line that answers the question (severity in this case) according to their evaluation. The value for their answer is obtained as the distance (cm) from the left end of the scale to the mark made. In this example the mark has been made one quarter up from 'best possible health'. Therefore if the VAS total length is 10 cm then the value for this example would be 2.5 cm.

The crucial aspect of this outcome measure is defining adequate 'anchor points', that is, values that reflect the extreme options available. This VAS was used to obtain parental and nurse assessment of severity of illness. A similar scale was used for GPs, but the anchors were 'child with a simple cold' and 'child sufficiently unwell to need admission to hospital'.

The CARIFS score is an example of a psychometric instrument; that is, it is a checklist of different items (fever, cough, appetite, irritability, etc.) that parents have to grade (0, 1, 2 or 3) according to the level that each of these items has been a problem. For example, if a mother sees her child with very high fevers but sleeping properly, she would rate Fever as level 3 whereas Sleep will get level 0. The sum of all these items is equal to the CARIFS score.

This scale can be thought of as having three different dimensions – symptoms, parental impact and function – each composed of five different items.

Symptoms	Parental impact	Function
Fever	Extra care	Interest
Cough	Clingy	Appetite
Nasal congestion	Crying	Irritable
Vomit	In bed	Energy
Unwell	Sleep	Play

The values for the total score range between 0 and 45 because each item can get a score between 0 and 3 and there are 15 in total.

Correlation coefficient (Pearson and Spearman)

The correlation coefficient (usually referred to as simply 'correlation') measures the degree of **linear association** between two variables. What this means is that if two variables (measured on the same individual) have the property that as one increases the other one does as well (for example, temperature and pulse rate) then these two will be **positively correlated**. By contrast, if when one of these increases the other one decreases then they will be **negatively correlated**. Finally if when one increases we cannot say what will happen to the other one (increase OR decrease) then these are not correlated.

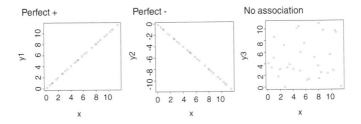

Generally there is variability in the measurement of the two variables so a perfect association is almost impossible to get. The correlation then measures how strong is the trend of the measurements falling close (or far) to a perfect line. The tighter they are to the line, the greater the correlation will be. In the extreme case – when all measurements fall on the line – the correlation will get a value of 1 (–1 if it is negative). When the values fall in such a way that a line is useless at describing the association between these variables then the correlation will be 0. This case could happen because there is no association – in which case we say that the variables are **independent** to each other (the value of one variable tells you nothing about the value of the other) – or because the association is not linear.

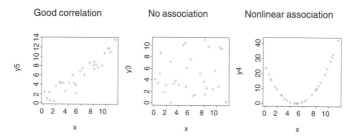

There are several coefficients that can be used to measure this association. The two most commonly used are the Pearson product moment correlation and the Spearman rank correlation.

The **Pearson correlation coefficient** is a parametric statistic, which means that the assumption behind this measurement is that the data are normally distributed. When this assumption is met, this statistic is the most useful way to measure the linear association between two variables, and it has a direct link with the coefficient obtained from using a linear regression to model the value of one variable from the other.

Spearman's rank correlation coefficient (often referred to as ρ (rho)) is a nonparametric statistic, which means that no assumption about the underlying distribution of the variables is made. It is also more robust than Pearson's correlation coefficient to a lack of linear association. This is because the association is not checked on the original values but on the ranks of those values (see rank tests). So as long as there is an increase in both variables (or increase in one and decrease in the other) it will detect an association even if this increase is not constant. Due to this, it can be used even when the variables being studied are categorical ordinal and obviously when they are continuous (and not normally distributed).

Interpretation: As mentioned above, when there is perfect association the values for the correlation are 1 (positive association) or −1 (negative). When no association is present the correlation will be equal to 0. As these are the extreme cases, generally a correlation coefficient (both Spearman and Pearson) will fall within the range of −1 to 1.

There is no clear consensus as to what is a high (low) correlation because this depends entirely on the context in which the correlation is being measured. Cohen (1988; see below) proposed the following values as anchors for interpretation in psychological research:

Correlation	Negative	Positive
Small	−0.29 to −0.10	0.10 to 0.29
Medium	−0.49 to −0.30	0.30 to 0.49
Large	−1.00 to −0.50	0.50 to 1.00

Use: Correlations are normally used to test if two variables are associated with each other. In this study, the main aim was to determine if parental measure of severity of illness was associated with that made by a health care worker (GP and nurse). Measuring the correlation will give an indication of how strong this association is.

Hypothesis testing: Many studies that measure correlation test the hypothesis that the correlation is equal to zero. If such a hypothesis was true, it would mean that the two variables have no linear association whatsoever and are therefore regarded as being independent (although this does not rule out other types of association that are not linear). One thing to notice about this approach is that it does not say anything about how great this correlation is, but just that it is significantly different from zero.

In this study, illness severity was measured using four different scales – GP VAS, Nurse VAS, Parent VAS and CARIFS.

	CARIFS					
	Overall	P. impact	Function	Symptom	GP VAS	Nurse VAS
GP VAS	0.13	0.09	0.03	0.16	–	–
Nurse VAS	0.35	0.20	0.38	0.36	0.24	–
Parent VAS	0.40	0.29	0.36	0.41	0.09	0.23

Spearman rank correlations

The highest correlation between these scores was between the Parent VAS and the CARIFS score (symptom dimension and overall score). This should be expected because both measurements were done by the same parent and they are aiming to measure the same thing (severity). However, it is of note that even then, this correlation is not particularly high, and using Cohen interpretation it would only fall into the medium association category. The interpretation of this could be that these two measures are not exactly measuring the same thing, hence the moderate association.

Also notable is that the smallest correlations are between parental scores (CARIFS and VAS) and GP VAS. In fact, a test of hypothesis (H_0: correlation is equal to 0) was nonsignificant (P value > 0.05). This would mean that from this dataset we could say that the severity measured by the parent (in either form) has no association to that measured by the GP.

Factor analysis and Cronbach's alpha

Factor analysis is a technique employed to reduce the number of variables being used while at the same time keeping most of the variability observed. It achieves this by creating new factors that are linear combinations of the measured variables plus error terms – similar to linear regression for each factor created. In this way one factor might include several (3, 4, etc.) variables reducing the total number in the analysis.

This technique groups interrelated variables and is commonly used to interpret results based on these factors. The CARIFS scale was created in such a way that three different factors are being measured – symptoms present, functional impact and parental burden. Each one of these factors is represented by five different items:

Symptom = Fever + Cough + Nasal congestion + Vomit + Unwell
Function = Interest + Appetite + Irritable + Energy + Play
Parent impact = Extra care + Clingy + Crying + In bed + Sleep

In creating a scale, there is a need for a strong overlap between the different items that form each factor. This redundancy is necessary because individuals' perceptions of one factor are variable. For example, one parent might find the extra care more problematic, whereas for another parent the opposite might be true in terms of how their sleep is being affected.

This redundancy can also be thought as a form of internal consistency (measuring the same thing). Cronbach's alpha is a commonly used measure of internal consistency, and its useful values range between 0 and 1 (highest). Cronbach's alpha will generally increase when the correlations between the items increase, and therefore it is closely related to factor analysis.

In practice, a scale with low alpha (less than 0.6) does not have adequate internal consistency; that is, the items in the scale are not measuring the same latent trait. On the other hand, very large values of alpha (over 0.9) point towards redundancy; that is, some items are not really needed. Several statistical packages can calculate this statistic, both for the overall scale and when reducing the scale by one item at a time. The latter procedure is very helpful in deciding which item to exclude when redundancy is suspected.

Scale dimension	alpha
Overall	0.85
Symptom	0.54
Function	0.77
Parent impact	0.70

The interpretation of this is that the overall scale has good internal consistency and could be regarded as a measure of overall severity. For each specific dimension, the internal consistency is adequate for function and parent impact; however, it is below what would be considered adequate for the symptom dimension.

A full description of factor analysis is beyond the scope of this book, but can be found mainly in books that deal with multivariate analysis techniques, such as Norman and Streiner (2000).

Cohen J. *Statistical Power Analysis for the Behavioral Sciences,* 2nd edn. Hillsdale, NJ: Lawrence Erlbaum Associates, 1988.

Norman GR, Streiner DL. *Biostatistics: The Bare Essentials,* 2nd edn. Hamilton, Ontario: BC Decker, 2000.

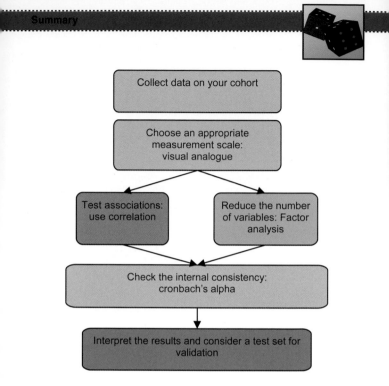

Statistical toolkit: Glossary

Absolute risk: the excess risk due to exposure to a hazard.

Absolute risk reduction (ARR): the difference in the event rate between the treated group (EER) and the control group (CER):

$$ARR = EER - CER$$

Adjustment: a summarising procedure for a statistical measure in which the effects of differences in composition of the populations being compared have been minimised by statistical methods.

Alpha value: a threshold level indicating the probability of accepting the alternative hypothesis when, in reality, the null hypothesis is true.

ANCOVA (analysis of covariance): a merger of regression and ANOVA; it tests for the effect of factors (ANOVA) after removing the effect accounted for by certain covariates (usually recorded at baseline).

ANOVA (analysis of variance): a group of statistical techniques used to compare the means of two or more samples to see whether they come from the same population. If more than one independent variable is tested, the approach is called a two-way ANOVA.

Association: an association occurs when two variables are related. Do not confuse association with causation: the relationship results from interaction or dependence.

Attributable risk: the rate of disease occurrence or death in a group that is exposed to a particular factor that can be attributed to the exposure to that factor. The term is sometimes incorrectly used to denote population attributable risk.

Bar chart: a chart used to summarise graphically and display the differences between groups of data.

Bell curve: the shape of the graph that indicates the normal (or related) distribution(s).

Beta coefficient (regression): beta is calculated using regression analysis, and is the change in the dependent variable (outcome) as the independent variable (factor) moves up one unit, everything else staying constant.

Beta statistic (power calculation): the probability of failing to reject the null hypothesis when it is false and a specific alternative hypothesis is true.

Bimodal distribution: a distribution with two different modes.

Bland–Altman plot: a statistical method to compare two measurement techniques. In this graphical method the differences (or alternatively the ratios) between the two techniques are plotted against the averages of the two techniques.

Bonferroni adjustment: a multiple-comparison correction used when several dependent or independent statistical tests are being performed simultaneously.

Bootstrapping: a statistical method that uses simulations to obtain estimates of the sampling distribution. Commonly used to calculate confidence limits of statistics that are not normally distributed.

Box plots: a graphical tool that displays the centre, spread and distribution of a continuous dataset, also known as **box and whisker diagram**.

Categorical variables: (sometimes called a nominal variable) a variable that has two or more categories, but without intrinsic ordering to the categories.

Censor data: occurs in survival analysis due to incomplete information on the outcome.

Centile or percentile: a number based on dividing something into 100 parts based on their frequency.

Chi-squared (test and distribution): a test that can be used to analyse the relationship between two categorised variables. Also a distribution derived from the normal distribution allowing the determination of whether actual frequencies in the data differ from frequencies that were expected.

Cluster analysis: a technique for the grouping of objects for which there are measurements of several variables.

Cluster data: a group of relatively homogeneous cases or observations.

Coefficient of variation: the standard deviation expressed as a percentage of the mean:

$$SD/\mu$$

The coefficient of variation (CV) indicates the quality of a population estimate. Estimates with either a moderate or high CV should be interpreted with caution. In some situations, the sample in the survey is too small to produce a reliable estimate.

Conditional probability: *see* probability.

Confidence interval (CI): the range around a study's result within which we would expect the true value to lie. CIs account for the sampling error between the sample and the population the study is supposed to represent (for a proportion):

$$P - \left[1.96 \times \sqrt{\frac{p(1-p)}{n}} \right] \quad \text{to} \quad P + \left[1.96 \times \sqrt{\frac{p(1-p)}{n}} \right]$$

Confounding variable: a variable that you may or may not be interested in but that affects the results of your trial.

Contingency table: a table (usually two rows and two columns) that is often used in epidemiology to show the relationship between disease and exposure:

	Disease (+ve)	Disease (−ve)
Exposed	a	c
Not exposed	b	d

Continuous variable: a variable that can take any value within a given range, for instance height, blood pressure, blood sugar.

Correlation: the strength and direction of a linear relationship between two random variables.

Cox regression: a method for investigating the effect of several variables upon the time a specified event takes to happen.

Cronbach's alpha: used for items in a scale to test that they are all measuring the same thing, i.e. they are correlated with one another.

Degrees of freedom: a measure of the number of independent pieces of information on which the precision of a parameter estimate is based.

Descriptive statistics: used to describe the basic features of data: a summary about the sample and the measures.

Determinant: any definable factor that effects a change in a health condition or other characteristic.

Discrete variable: a variable that can only be given as certain values, normally whole numbers, e.g. children in a given family.

EER: experimental event rate; *see* Event rate.

Effect size: a generic term for the estimate of effect for a study. A dimensionless measure of effect that is typically used for continuous data when different scales (e.g. for measuring depression) are used to measure an outcome. It is usually defined as the difference in means between the intervention and control groups divided by the standard deviation of the control or both groups.

Error: the amount an observation differs from its true value.

Event rate: the proportion of patients in a group in whom an event is observed:

$$Er = n/d$$

n = numerator
d = denominator

Factor analysis: a statistical technique used to estimate factors or to reduce the dimensionality of a number of variables to a few factors.

F distribution: a continuous probability distribution, also known as the Fisher–Snedecor distribution.

Fisher's exact test: used to determine if there are nonrandom associations between two categorical variables. It is used for data in a two-by-two contingency table. Such a table arises in a variety of contexts, most often when a new therapy is compared with a standard therapy and the outcome measure is binary. Use Fisher's exact test in situations where a large sample approximation is inappropriate.

Fixed effect model: a model used in meta-analysis to assess the level of uncertainty (confidence interval) that takes into account within-study sampling and not the between study variation.

Forest plot: a diagrammatic representation of the results of individual trials in a meta-analysis.

Frequencies: the measurement of the number of times that a repeated event occurs per unit time:

$$F = x/t$$

x = repeated event
t = unit time

Funnel plot: a method of graphing the results of trials in a meta-analysis to show if the results have been affected by publication bias.

Hazard ratio (HR): the ratio of the hazard (harmful event) in one group of observations divided by the hazard of an event in a different group.

Heterogeneity: in systematic reviews, the amount of incompatibility between trials included in the review, whether clinical (i.e. the studies are clinically different), methodological (i.e. different study designs) or statistical (i.e. the results are different from one another).

Histogram: a block graph with no spaces between the blocks. It is used to represent frequency data in statistics.

Homogeneity: in systematic reviews, the amount of compatibility between trials included in the review, whether clinical (i.e. the studies are clinically similar or comparable) or statistical (i.e. the results are similar to one another).

Hypothesis: a testable statement that predicts the relationship between two variables.

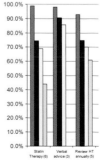

Incidence: the number of new cases of illness arising, or of persons falling ill, during a specified time period in a given population.

Intention-to-treat: characteristic of a study where patients are analysed in the groups to which they were originally assigned, even though they may have switched treatment arms during the study for clinical reasons.

Interaction effects: the effects of a factor averaged over another factor.

Interclass correlation coefficient: used to assess the degree of resemblance between two members of different classes with respect to a specified characteristic.

Interval variable: is similar to an ordinal variable, except that the intervals between the values of the interval variable are equally spaced.

Intraclass correlation coefficient: used to assess the degree of resemblance among members of the same class with respect to a specified characteristic.

Kaplan–Meier (survival plot): a graphical method to display a sample cohort's survival: the survival estimates are recalculated whenever there is a death.

Kappa: The measure of the level of agreement between two categorical measures.

Value of kappa	Strength of agreement
<0.20	Poor
0.21–0.40	Fair
0.41–0.60	Moderate
0.61–0.80	Good
0.81–1.00	Very good

Linear regression: the relation between variables when the regression equation is linear:

$$y = ax + b$$

Log-rank test: a method for comparing two survival curves.

Mean: the average value in a sample.

Meta-analysis: the use of quantitative methods to summarise the results of several studies. Often used as a synonym for systematic reviews; however, not all systematic reviews contain a meta-analysis.

Meta-regression: can be considered as an extension to meta-analysis that can be used to investigate the heterogeneity of effects across studies. It examines the relationship between one or more study-level characteristics and the sizes of effect observed in the studies.

Missing data: part of almost all research, and one that demands a decision on how to deal with the problem.

Mode: the most frequent value of a random variable.

Multiple comparisons: performance of multiple analyses on the same data. There is an increased chance of a type I error.

Multiple regression: an analysis where two or more independent (predictor) variables affect the dependent variable.

Multivariate analysis: statistical methods for analysing more than two variables simultaneously.

Negative predictive value (−PV): the proportion of people with a negative test who are free of disease.

Nonproportional hazard: used when the hazard ratio is not constant over time.

Normal distribution: data distribution simulating a bell-shaped curve that is symmetrical around the mean so that the data exhibit an equal chance of being above or below the mean.

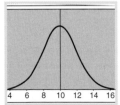

Null hypothesis (H_0): a hypothesis that there is no difference between the two intervention groups being tested. The result either rejects or does not reject the hypothesis (with a certain probability of error).

Number needed to treat (NNT): the average number of patients who need to be treated to prevent one bad outcome. It is the inverse of the ARR:

$$NNT = 1/ARR$$

Odds: the ratio of the number of times an event happens to the number of times it does not happen in a group of patients.
If 10 people have a heart attack out of 100 in the intervention group the odds are 10/90 = 1:9.

Odds ratio: the odds of an event happening in one group divided by the odds in a different group.

One-way analysis of variance: *see* ANOVA.

Ordinal: an ordinal variable is similar to a categorical variable. The difference between the two is that there is ordering of the categories.

Outliers: observations that deviate from or fall considerably outside most of the other scores or observations in a distribution or pattern.

Paired samples: two measurements are said to be paired when they come from the same observational unit. When they do not come from the same unit observations are paired when there is a natural link between an observation in one set of measurements and a particular observation in the other set of measurements, irrespective of their actual values.

Parametric techniques: tests that make certain assumptions:
1. The data are drawn from a normal – or other specific – distribution.
2. The data are measured on an interval scale.
3. Parametric tests generally make use of parameters such as the mean and standard deviation.

Partial correlation: the correlation between two variables with the influence of a third variable statistically controlled for.

Pearson correlation: a measure of the correlation of two (interval) variables *a* and *b* measured on the same object.

Population attributable risk: is different from the attributable risk in that it estimates the proportion of disease in the study population that is attributable to exposure to a specific risk factor. In order to calculate it, the incidence of exposure in the study population must be known or estimated.

Positive predictive value (+PV): the proportion of people with a positive test who have the disease.

Post hoc analysis: analysing the data after the end of the trial for results that were not pre-specified.

Post-test probability: the probability that a patient has the disorder of interest after the test result is known.

Power calculation: an estimation of the ability of a study to provide a result rejecting the null hypothesis with a given measure of precision.

Pre-test probability: the probability that a patient has the disorder of interest prior to administering a test.

Prevalence: the total number of observations in a population at a given time. Typically expressed as a percentage.

Probability: a measure that quantifies the uncertainty associated with an event. If an event A cannot happen the probability p(A) is 0; if an event happens with certainty the probability p(A) is 1. All others outcomes and values lie between these two variables. Probabilities can also be expressed as percentages. **Conditional probability** is the probability that event A occurs given event B, usually written p(A|B). An example is the probability of a positive faecal occult blood test given a diagnosis of colon cancer. Be careful not to get confused: the probability of A and B is not the same as the probability of A given B.

Proportional hazard (Cox's proportional hazard): used to estimate the effects of different covariates influencing the times-to-event.

_P_ value: the probability that a particular result or some more extreme (if the H_0 is correct) would have happened by chance.

Quartile: a segment of a sample representing a sequential quarter (25%) of the group.

Random effects: a model used in meta-analysis to estimate a pooled effect that takes into account both within-study sampling error and between-studies variation. If there is significant heterogeneity random effects models will give wider confidence intervals than fixed effect models.

Range: limits of the values a function or variable can take.

Rank: the position of an observation in the sequence of sample values arranged in order, usually from lowest to highest.

Receiver operating characteristic curve (ROC curve): a graphical plot of sensitivity versus 1 – specificity.

Recode: to transform information into a different code.

Regression: statistical modelling that attempts to evaluate the relationship between one variable – the dependent variable – and one or more other variables – the independent variables.

Regression analysis: the use of regression to make quantitative predictions of one variable from the values of another.

Regression dilution: statistical variability in the predictor variable x leads to bias in the estimate of the gradient (slope) of the regression line.

Regression to the mean: the tendency of a random variable that is distinct from the norm to return to the mean value and the impact of this in the regression estimates (usually reducing the effect).

Relative risk (RR) (or risk ratio): the ratio of the risk of an event in the experimental group compared with that of the control group. Not to be confused with relative risk reduction (see below).

$$RR = EER/CER$$

Relative risk reduction (RRR): the percentage reduction in events in the treated group event rate (EER) compared with the control group event rate (CER):

$$RRR = (EER - CER)/CER$$

Residual: an observable **estimate** of the unobservable error.

Risk: the probability that an event will occur for a particular patient or group of patients. Risk can be expressed as a decimal fraction or percentage (e.g. 0.25 or 25%).

Sample size: the number of patients studied in a trial, including the treatment and control groups. A larger sample size decreases the probability of making a false-positive error and increases the power of a trial.

Scatter-plot: a two-dimensional graph representing a set of bivariate data: for each element being graphed, there are two separate pieces of data.

Sensitivity of a diagnostic test: the proportion of people with disease who have a positive test.

Significance level (alpha): the probability of rejecting a set of assumptions when they are in fact true.

Significance testing: tests used to determine whether the observed difference between sample proportions could occur by chance in the populations from which the samples were selected.

Sign test: a test based on the sign of a difference between two related observations. Usually a plus sign (+) is used for a positive difference between observations and a minus sign (–) for a negative difference between observations.

Skewness: a probability distribution that shows a lack of symmetry about the mean, or any measure of the lack of symmetry.

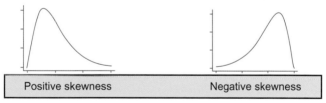

Positive skewness   Negative skewness

Spearman correlation: a nonparametric measure of correlation used to describe the relationship between two variables, without making any assumptions about the frequency distribution of the variables.

Specificity of a diagnostic test: the proportion of people free of a disease who have a negative test.

Standard deviation (SD): a measure of the spread or deviation of values from the mean. The standard deviation is the positive square root of the variance and is depicted by s for samples, or by σ for populations.

> **For a normal distribution**
> **1 SD includes 68.2% of the variables**
> **2 SD includes 95.4%**
> **3 SD includes 99.7%**

Standard error (SE): the standard deviation of the sampling distribution of the mean. The SE is calculated by dividing the standard deviation of the sample by the square root of the number of subjects in the sample:

$$SE = SD/\sqrt{n}$$

Stratification: a process of grouping data according to a common characteristic.

Subgroup analysis: an analysis of treatment effects in different types of patient in order to decide who will benefit most from being given the treatment.

Survival analysis: statistical analysis that evaluates the timing of death occurring in a cohort over time.

Survival curve: a graph of the number of events occurring over time or the chance of being free of these events over time. The events must be discrete and the time at which they occur must be precisely known. In most clinical situations, the chance of an outcome changes with time. In most survival curves the earlier follow-up periods usually include results from more patients than the later periods and are therefore more precise.

Tailed tests: a **one-tailed test** is where the null hypothesis can only be rejected in one direction – e.g. if a new intervention is worse than current intervention but not better. A **two-tailed test** is where the null hypothesis can be rejected whether the new intervention is better or worse than the control or current intervention.

Hence, a one-tailed test looks for an increase (or decrease) in the parameter whereas a two-tailed test looks for any change in the parameter (both increase or decrease).

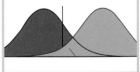

Test-retest reliability: a measure of the reliability obtained by giving individuals the same test for a second time after an interval and correlating the scores.

Test statistic: the summary value of a dataset that is compared with a statistical distribution to determine whether the dataset differs from that expected under a null hypothesis.

Transformation: a change in the size, shape, location or orientation of a figure.

Type I error: the chance of rejecting the null hypothesis when it is actually true (false positive).

Type II error: the chance of not rejecting the null hypothesis when it is actually false (false negative).

Uniform distribution: a distribution in which all possible outcomes have an equal chance of occurring.

Validity: (in psychometrics) whether or not a test measures what it was designed to measure; (in research design) whether or not a study's results support the conclusions.

Variance: a measure of the spread of scores away from the mean. It is the square of the standard deviation.

Variation: the amount of change or difference from expected results.

Weighted average: an average that has been adjusted to allow for the relative importance of the data.

Weighted mean or weighted mean difference: in meta-analysis, information for continuous variables measures can be combined using the mean, standard deviation and sample size in each group. The weight given to each study (how much influence each study has on the overall results of the meta-analysis) is determined by the precision of the study's estimate of effect and, in the statistical software RevMan, is equal to the inverse of the variance. This method assumes that all of the trials have measured the outcome on the same scale.

Wilcoxon (paired/unpaired) signed rank test: a nonparametric test for comparing two related samples or repeated measurements on a single sample.

Yates' continuity correction: used when testing for independence in a contingency table. It requires the assumption that the discrete probability of observed frequencies can be approximated by the chi-squared distribution, which is continuous.

z statistic: used for inference procedures on the population mean.

Software for data management and statistical analysis

There are numerous and different types of software packages available for data management and statistical analysis. However, with some basic understanding of the statistical methods, and particularly of the assumptions required for each, it is relatively easy to switch from one statistical package to another.

Invariably, data management and statistical analysis are interrelated. Due to this, most of the statistical software packages will have functions and methods for data management such as displaying data, adding or editing variables or data, and data manipulation (e.g. transforming variables). At the same time, data management software usually has some basic statistical methods integrated (e.g. calculation of basic descriptive statistics).

Microsoft Excel is an example of a highly flexible package that allows you to do most of the data management easily. However, it has severe limitations when the dataset involved is relatively large; moreover the statistical methods on offer are limited.

	Microsoft Excel - Book3					
File Edit View Insert Format Tools Data Window Help Adobe PDF						
G3		fx =AVERAGE(E2:E327)				
	A	B	C	D	E	F	G
1	idno	group	withdraw	cured2	daycure		
2	A1	1	0	1	6		
3	A10	1	0	1	4		3.756272
4	A11	2	0	1	1		
5	A12	2	0	1	3		
6	A13	2	0	1	5		
7	A14	1	0	1	2		
8	A15	1	0	1	6		

You can select a variable and move it into the Label Cases by box: numeric or string. Commands can be used to calculate statistics such as means (average), medians (median), standard deviations (stdev), etc.

To view the different (simple) statistical methods available a click at the *fx* icon while selecting Statistical as category would give a list of these.

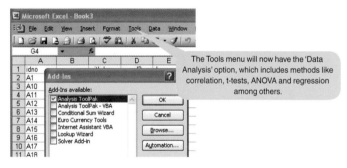

More complex statistical methods can be accessed using the Data Analysis Toolpack, which needs to be activated by using the Add-ins options in the Tools menu.

There are only a handful of statistical methods available through Microsoft Excel, and the maximum size of database is restricted to 65 536 rows × 256 columns. For most applications in medicine this space is enough, which means that Excel is the preferred package when creating databases that are then transferred to a dedicated statistical software like SPSS, STATA, SAS or R (to name a few).

For this reason some statistical packages have 'filters' that will allow a direct translation from Excel into their own format, while others will translate .txt files generated in Excel. This is done by saving the Excel file as a Tab delimited text file.

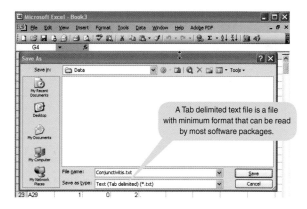

A Tab delimited text file is a file with minimum format that can be read by most software packages.

Each statistical software package has its own advantages, for example SPSS is relatively simple to manage and use. STATA is slightly less intuitive, but has many extra methods available as part of the basic package. SAS and R are probably the less intuitive out of the four mentioned here. SAS has the advantage of handling very large databases optimally, whereas R allows the user total control on the creation of graphs. For this reason we limit this section only to show how to import a dataset and do a basic analysis of it using SPSS and STATA.

SPSS is a very intuitive package that allows the user to analyse data with the minimum of confusion. It is excellent for basic analysis and for some slightly less basic ones. This package has an internal filter that allows an Excel file to be imported directly into SPSS.

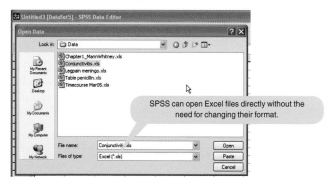

SPSS can open Excel files directly without the need for changing their format.

[SPSS Data Editor screenshot with Analyze menu expanded]

All statistical methods appear under one heading in the menu – Analyze. The basic exploratory statistics can be calculated using the Descriptive Statistics, as well as many of the basic graphical displays such as histograms, pie charts, bar charts, etc.

Pallant J. *SPSS Survival Manual*, 2nd edn. Open University Press.

[SPSS Data Editor screenshot showing the Frequencies dialog box]

The Frequencies menu has many options to select the best way of displaying and exploring the data such as histograms and bar charts, as well as being able to provide central tendency (mean, median, etc.) and dispersion measures (standard deviation, interquartile range, etc.).

STATA is an intermediate package in the sense that it is still intuitive enough to use without needing to spend much effort in understanding the commands used, while at the same time still being used by researchers of statistics to develop new methods that are then made available to the community of STATA users.

To import a database generated in Excel into STATA this database needs to have been saved as a Tab delimited text file in Excel in the first place. This file can then be accessed using the Import option in STATA.

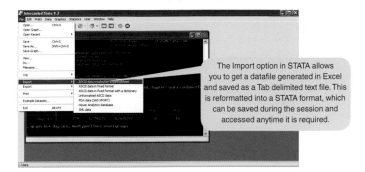

The Import option in STATA allows you to get a datafile generated in Excel and saved as a Tab delimited text file. This is reformatted into a STATA format, which can be saved during the session and accessed anytime it is required.

As with SPSS, STATA can be menu driven – both have the option to use commands instead, but this application is beyond the limits of this book. For STATA, the statistical methods available appear under the Statistics menu. The basic exploratory methods can be found under the Summaries subheading within the Summaries, tables & tests heading.

In contrast with SPSS, there are several windows that can be on display at the same time in STATA. These are: Results, Command, Graph, Viewer, Variables, Review and Data editor. It can take some time to get used to them, particularly because the appearance of one of these windows can trigger the disappearance of another one (e.g. when the Data editor appears, the Command window is not available).

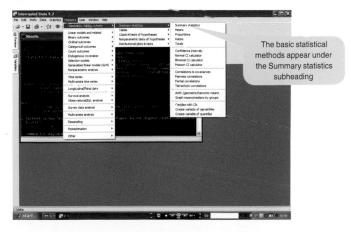

The basic statistical methods appear under the Summary statistics subheading

References

Doust JA, Pietrzak E, Dobson A, Glasziou P. How well does B-type natriuretic peptide predict death and cardiac events in patients with heart failure: systematic review. *Br Med J* 2005;**330**(7492):625. PMID: 15774989.

Harnden A, Brueggemann A, Shepperd S *et al.* Near patient testing for influenza in children in primary care: comparison with laboratory test. *Br Med J* 2003;**326**(7387):480. PMID: 12609945.

Harnden A, Ninis N, Thompson M *et al.* Parenteral penicillin for children with meningococcal disease before hospital admission: case-control study. Br Med J 2006;**332**(7553):1295–8. PMID: 16554335.

Heneghan C, Alonso-Coello P, Garcia-Alamino JM *et al.* Self-monitoring of oral anticoagulation: a systematic review and meta-analysis. *Lancet* 2006;**367**(9508):404–11. PMID: 16458764.

Johansson JE, Andrén O, Andersson SO *et al.* Natural history of early, localized prostate cancer.*JAMA* 2004;**291**(22):2713–19. PMID: 15187052.

Rose PW, Harnden A, Brueggemann AB *et al.* Chloramphenicol treatment for acute infective conjunctivitis in children in primary care: a randomised double-blind placebo-controlled trial. *Lancet* 2005;**366**(9479):37–43. PMID: 15993231.

Shepperd S, Perera R, Bates S *et al.* A children's acute respiratory illness scale (CARIFS) predicted functional severity and family burden. *J Clin Epidemiol* 2004;**57**(8):809–14. PMID: 15485733.

Shepperd S, Farndon P, Grainge V *et al.* DISCERN-Genetics: quality criteria for information on genetic testing. *Eur J Hum Genet* 2006;**14**(11):1179–88. PMID: 16868557.

Thompson MJ, Ninis N, Perera R *et al.* Clinical recognition of meningococcal disease in children and adolescents. *Lancet* 2006;**367**(9508):397–403. PMID: 16458763.

Index